Gastrointestinal Endoscopy
Beyond the Basics

Provided as an
educational service by:

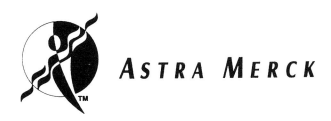

ASTRA MERCK

Gastrointestinal Endoscopy

Beyond the Basics

John Baillie, B.Sc.(Hons), M.B. Ch.B., F.R.C.P.(Glasg), F.A.C.G.

Associate Professor of Medicine and Director,
Hepatobiliary and Pancreatic Disorders Service,
Division of Gastroenterology, Duke University Medical Center,
Durham, North Carolina

Butterworth–Heinemann
Boston   Oxford   Johannesburg   Melbourne   New Delhi   Singapore

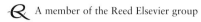
 Recognizing the importance of preserving what has been written, Butterworth–Heinemann prints its books on acid-free paper whenever possible.

Library of Congress Cataloging-in-Publication Data
Baillie, John, FRCP (Glasg.)
    Gastrointestinal endoscopy : beyond the basics / John Baillie.
        p.   cm.
    "A sequel to: Gastrointestinal endoscopy : basic principles and practice"--Pref.
    Includes bibliographical references and index.
    ISBN 0-7506-9555-2
    1. Endoscopy.   2. Gastrointestinal system--Diseases--Diagnosis.
    I. Title.
      [DNLM: 1. Endoscopy, Gastrointestinal--methods.
    2. Gastrointestinal Diseases--diagnosis.   3. Gastrointestinal
    Diseases--therapy. WI 141 B157g 1997]
    RC804.E6B352   1997
    616.3'307545--dc21
    DNLM/DLC
    for Library of Congress   96-50473
                                                                           CIP

British Library Cataloguing-in-Publication Data
A catalogue record for this book is available from the British Library.

The publisher offers special discounts on bulk orders of this book.
For information, please contact:

Manager of Special Sales
Butterworth–Heinemann
313 Washington Street
Newton, MA 02158–1626
Tel: 617-928-2500
Fax: 617-928-2620

For information on all B-H medical publications available, contact our World Wide Web home page at: http://www.bh.com/med

10 9 8 7 6 5 4 3 2

Printed in the United States of America

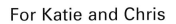
For Katie and Chris

Contents

Preface

This book is a sequel to *Gastrointestinal Endoscopy: Basic Principles and Practice*. It is intended to add breadth and depth to a variety of subjects. The technology and techniques of gastrointestinal (GI) endoscopy continue to undergo very rapid evolution. Therefore, I have tried to provide up-to-date views on each technology and application where possible. In the 5 years since *Gastrointestinal Endoscopy: Basic Principles and Practice* was published, small-bowel enteroscopy has undergone considerable development and therefore merits a section of its own. Similarly, endoscopic ultrasound (EUS) continues to grow and find broad applications in expert hands. Some may consider my coverage of EUS too superficial. However, it is a highly specialized technique with a long learning curve that requires in-depth study and training. I offer simply a "snapshot" to whet the serious student's appetite. My trainees have frequently complained that information regarding the physics and tissue effects of laser is hard to find. I have attempted to fill this void. The use of laser technology in the GI tract is expanding, with photodynamic therapy for tumors and Barrett's esophagus and new delivery systems such as the contact laser and water-guided laser system. In Chapter 2 I describe some of the ingenious techniques that have been developed to tackle difficult problems in the colon, including resection techniques for large polyps, ways to identify early cancers (which are often sessile), marking polyp resection sites with India ink, and laser fluorescence to identify dysplasia. Finally, this book explores some more complex issues in endoscopic retrograde cholangiopancreatography and discusses new and evolving endoscopic technology.

As with *Gastrointestinal Endoscopy: Basic Principles and Practice*, this book is not intended to be encyclopedic. Detailed descriptions of the techniques can be found in published reports in the specialist journals [e.g., *Gastrointestinal Endoscopy*] and in the larger textbooks of endoscopy. It is fair to say that for many of the problems discussed, there is no "right way" to perform the diagnostic or therapeutic procedure. While there is room for many variations on a basic theme, there are certain safety issues that should always be considered. I encourage readers to review the guidelines of the American Society of Gastrointestinal Endoscopy for the use of endoscopic procedures. These guidelines have been formulated by committees of expert endoscopists and represent a consensus on safe and acceptable practice. Endoscopists should be able to recognize and manage complications of their procedures. We are only now beginning to get an accurate picture of endoscopic complication rates from well-designed prospective studies. Prospective evaluation of complications provides a more realistic estimate of true complication rates, which are almost always higher than reported in retrospective studies.

I am indebted to many individuals for their encouragement, especially Dick Kozarek of Seattle, an old friend and mentor whose wise counsel has often kept me out of trouble. I am also grateful to many trainees and colleagues (too many to mention individually) who were kind enough to provide feedback after reading *Gastrointestinal Endoscopy: Basic Principles and Practice*. Their comments and suggestions have been incorporated into revisions of that book and have also shaped the style and content of the current text. I have been privileged to work with many fine endoscopists at Duke University, both faculty and fellows; I have learned something from each of them. Dr. Klaus Mergener, one of our rising stars at Duke, reviewed the manuscript of this textbook and offered many helpful suggestions. Two former fellows, who are now my partners, Drs. Stan Branch and Paul Jowell, have helped me in many ways and deserve special mention for their innovation and willingness to experiment. Our team of GI endoscopy nurses at Duke University Medical Center has provided support and encouragement over the last 8 years. Ann Hauman of Beaufort, North Carolina, provided the line drawings for this textbook. A relative newcomer to medical illustration, she has done a commendable job. I also thank Glen Hoskin of the Wilson-Cook Company (Winston-Salem, North Carolina) for generously making available to me photographs of many endoscopic accessories. The Medical Photography Department at Duke University Medical Center did its usual expert job of preparing the illustrations for dispatch to the publisher. It has been my great pleasure to work with the United States branch of Butterworth–Heinemann, especially Susan Pioli, Michelle St. Jean-Richards, and Jana Friedman. They have exhibited great patience and optimism during this project. Elizabeth Willingham and her team at Silverchair Science + Communications did a sterling job of preparing the book for publication and were a joy to work with. I also acknowledge the support of local representatives of Glaxo Pharmaceuticals who contributed toward the cost of the illustrations. I am especially indebted to my excellent secretary, Libby Honeycutt, for her expert assistance in preparing the manuscript. Dr. Rodger Liddle, Chief of the Division of Gastroenterology at Duke University Medical Center, has been very supportive of my educational activities, including the preparation of this book. Finally, thanks as always to my wife, Alison, and children, Katie and Christopher, for suffering through yet another book project.

J.B.

1

Upper Gastrointestinal Problems and Solutions

Difficult Esophageal Intubation

Aside from flexible sigmoidoscopy, upper gastrointestinal (GI) endoscopy (esophagogastroduodenoscopy [EGD]) is usually assumed to be the easiest of endoscopic procedures, and 95 times out of 100, this is true. However, the skilled endoscopist should have the experience to recognize the technically problematic intubation and deal with it accordingly. Inexperienced endoscopists often respond to difficulty with intubating the esophagus by pushing too hard, which inevitably causes trauma to a very sensitive area. At the very least, it is distressing to the patient and at worst, it may result in a perforation of the hypopharynx or upper esophagus. High perforations are especially difficult to manage and are to be avoided at all costs.

Can one predict which patients are likely to be difficult to intubate? Certainly, a history of prior difficulty passing an endoscope should be a red flag. All patients complaining of dysphagia should be approached with caution because their complaint may be due to a stenosis or other anatomic problem, such as a pharyngeal diverticulum. Patients who have recently ingested corrosives require particular care. Often, there is considerable edema and friability of the mucosa of the hypopharynx and esophagus following a chemical burn. This makes defining the anatomic landmarks more difficult and increases the potential for instrumental trauma. Patients who have had neck surgery for pharyngeal or laryngeal tumors often have altered anatomy. When performing EGD on these patients, it is mandatory to do it under direct vision. In my opinion, every EGD should be performed under direct vision because it not only makes the procedure safer but also increases the yield of pathology. There is little justification for routine blind intubation. It is frequently said that patients with marked osteoarthritis present a problem for intubation due to bone spurs protruding anteriorly from the cervical spine, impinging on the upper esophagus. In practice, this is rarely a problem now, presumably because of the smaller diameter of modern gastroscopes, but care should be taken to avoid forced extension or flexion of any arthritic patient's neck.

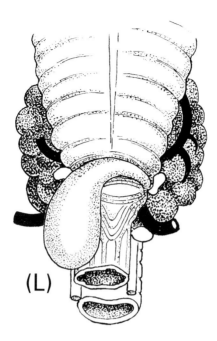

(L)

Figure 1-1. Posterior view of Zenker's diverticulum. The majority of these diverticula arise from the left side (L) of the hypopharynx.

Should every patient undergoing EGD for dysphagia have a contrast study performed first? This is an old argument but one that continues to raise considerable heat. I think it depends a great deal on the circumstances of the dysphagia. If a foreign body impaction is the anticipated cause, contrast radiology rarely adds much. Indeed, if barium is used, it can be difficult to see the food bolus (or whatever is causing the obstruction). Dysphagia or odynophagia in patients undergoing drug therapy (including immunosuppression) may be infective (e.g., *Candida*, cytomegalovirus) or related to the medication itself (e.g., nonsteroidal anti-inflammatory drugs, potassium, tetracycline). Contrast radiology adds nothing here. On the other hand, the information provided by contrast studies in patients with benign and malignant strictures can be most useful in planning management. Also, a Zenker's diverticulum (Figure 1-1) that might not otherwise be seen may be apparent on a barium study. Opinions on contrast radiology versus endoscopy tend to become polarized, but in fact these studies are complementary: There are situations in which both are useful. The study should be tailored to the indication.

Esophageal Strictures

When attempting to perform EGD in the presence of a suspected stricture or other anatomic abnormality, it is wise to have fluoroscopy (radiographic screening) available. Many endoscopy units now have C-arm–type mobile fluoroscopy units. Provided that the patient is on a cart designed to accommodate such a unit, fluoroscopy can be arranged at short notice. If the C-arm unit is not in the endoscopy room, it can be wheeled in and positioned within minutes. Where a mobile C-arm unit is not available, consideration should be given to starting the procedure with the patient lying on a dedicated fluoroscopy table. There are several benefits of fluoroscopy. First, it helps to define the position of the endoscope tip accurately. Second, it can be used to monitor guidewire placement for subsequent Savary-type dilation (CR Bard, Inc., Billerica, MA). Third, if tapered mercury dilators (e.g., Maloney [Medovations, Inc., Milwaukee, WI] and Hurst [Hurst, Research Triangle Park, NC]) are used, their progress can be monitored. The exception to the need for fluoroscopy is the stable, chronic, symmetric benign stricture, which may be safely dilated using weighted bougies. Indeed, many patients use these dilators at home without supervision.

If there is more than mild resistance to the advancement of a standard gastroscope, which on average is 9–11 mm in external diameter, then it should be withdrawn and consideration be given to an alternative approach. It is worth attempting to pass a pediatric-size endoscope, if available. The pediatric endoscope has the theoretical advantage of a small diameter, but in practice, it is somewhat cumbersome to use. It lacks the stiffness of the standard gastroscope insertion tube and has a small instrument channel, which severely limits the size of guidewires and accessories that can be used through it. The smaller-diameter endoscope allows inspection of the offending lesion (e.g., stricture, diverticulum).

If a small-diameter scope is not available, consider blind dilation of a presumed stricture. Some endoscopists would stop at this stage and arrange for a contrast study to delineate the abnormality prior to a repeat attempt. If fluoroscopy is available, however, many would carefully pass a guidewire to facilitate progressive dilation of the stricture. The position of the guidewire must be accurately monitored using fluoroscopy. Great care must be taken not to apply undue pressure to overcome resistance when passing the guidewire, otherwise local (contained) or free perforation may occur. This is of particular concern when dealing with malignant strictures. Usually, however, one can be reasonably sure that the guidewire has crossed the stricture and passed through the esophagus without problems. The tip is seen to coil in the stomach (Figure 1-2). Guidewires usually cause problems when they assume an acute angle, suggesting axial forces transmitted from the tip. Wires can break at these angles and cause perforation. As always in endoscopy, anything more than mild resistance to advancement is cause for great caution.

With the guidewire safely positioned and monitored by fluoroscopy, serial dilation with over-the-wire dilators can begin. The Savary-type plastic dilator is probably the most widely used today (Figure 1-3). One version of this dilator has been impregnated with barium to make it more radiopaque (Figure 1-4). The standard Savary dilator has markings near the tip and at

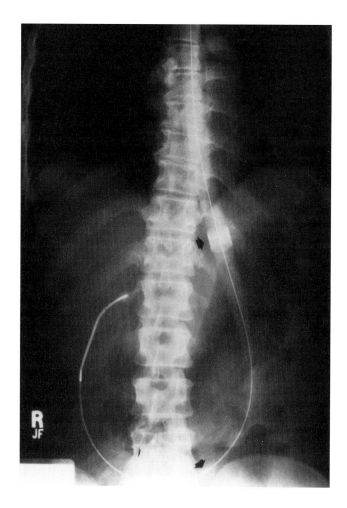

Figure 1-2. Fluoroscopic image of the tip of a Savary guidewire coiling in the stomach.

the waist to allow the endoscopist to determine when the stricture has been crossed. As always when dilating strictures, start small and work up, observing the rule of three: go to a maximum of the third dilator beyond the size at which initial resistance was encountered. The rule of three has become somewhat muddied because the diameter of newer dilators does not increase in a standard stepwise fashion. Therefore, the degree of dilation between serial dilators may be larger than in the past, when mercury dilators (e.g., Maloney) were used. High esophageal or hypopharyngeal strictures are often tight and so a dilator of small diameter is required. After serial dilation, it is often possible to advance a standard or pediatric-size endoscope.

Occasionally, it remains difficult to pass the endoscope after apparently successful dilatation. In this case, it is worth attempting to pass the endo-

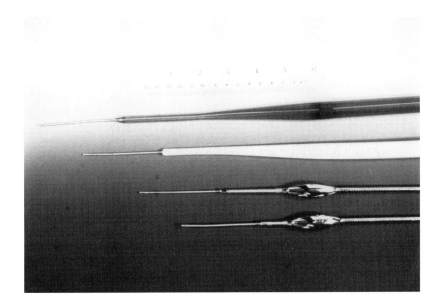

Figure 1-3. The new and the old: Savary-type plastic esophageal dilators (top two) and now (almost) obsolete olive (Eder-Puestow) dilators (lower two).

scope over the guidewire of the Savary kit, but the bare end of the wire should not be threaded into the endoscope instrument channel without protection because it is almost guaranteed to damage the rubber lining, necessitating an expensive repair. A plastic catheter, such as that used to cover guidewires during endoscopic retrograde cholangiopancreatography (ERCP) (an inner catheter), can be passed through the scope and the wire advanced (retrograde) through it. The catheter can then be advanced over the wire through the stricture or upper esophageal sphincter to protect it from trauma during attempted intubation. Using fluoroscopy to monitor the position of the guidewire–catheter, the endoscope can then be advanced (traction is required on the guidewire–catheter to prevent it advancing further than desired). This technique is often successful in getting the gastroscope through the narrowing. If there is no further need for the guidewire, the guidewire–catheter can be withdrawn through the endoscope and the endoscopy completed in the normal fashion. This guidewire–catheter intubation trick is equally helpful when difficulty is encountered passing a side-viewing scope for ERCP.

What should one do if the resistance met at the upper esophageal sphincter or upper esophagus remains significant even after attempted dilation? Provided that the patient does not have total aphagia, it may be safer to concede defeat and return another day to repeat the procedure. This is certainly a wise decision in the presence of a long, tight stricture, as may be seen in caustic or other corrosive injury. In such cases, regular dilation two or three times per week may be needed to get the

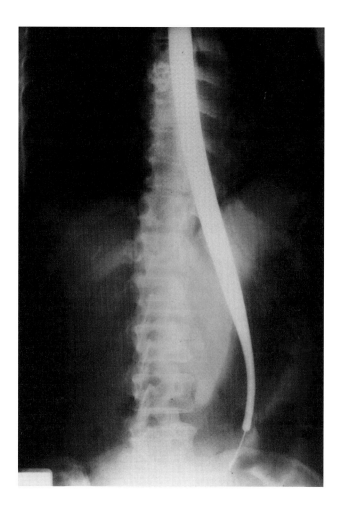

Figure 1-4. A barium-impregnated esophageal dilator is radiopaque on a fluoroscopic image.

lumen of the strictured area up to a diameter at which an endoscope can be safely passed. Of course, surgeons have long been familiar with the technique of retrograde dilation of tough esophageal strictures using dilators pulled up through a gastrostomy incision. Fortunately, advances in endoscopic technology have meant that recourse to such invasive measures is unusual.

Malignant strictures of the esophagus rarely stay open after endoscopic dilation. This is hardly surprising, given the rigidity of many of these strictures. Endoscopic intubation using a plastic or metal prosthesis is one means of palliating such strictures (see the section on Plastic Esophageal Prostheses). Other methods applied to malignant strictures include alcohol injection (which necroses the tumor) and laser and Bicap probes (Olympus Corp., Roswell, GA, or Boston Scientific Corp.,

Watertown, MA), all with the intention of restoring patency of the lumen. None of these methods is ideal, and all have their particular technical problems and risks. Because a few esophageal tumors respond to simple dilation alone, this is an approach worth taking when more aggressive methods are not available or the patient expresses a wish not to have these procedures performed. If regular dilation can be achieved by the patient at home using a mercury bougie or balloon dilator (Figure 1-5A and B), this may keep the patient swallowing saliva and able to maintain fluid intake. This is often adequate palliation in a terminally ill patient.

Dilation in the Presence of Esophageal Diverticula

The majority of esophageal diverticula are not true diverticula because they lack all the layers of the bowel wall. Accordingly, their correct designation would be *pseudodiverticula*. For the purposes of the following discussion, however, the term *diverticulum* (plural, *diverticula*) is used to describe this anatomic abnormality.

Esophageal diverticula used to be classified as *pulsion* and *traction*, according to their assumed etiology. Traction diverticula were thought to result from external forces on the esophageal wall, most commonly enlarged mediastinal lymph nodes in tuberculosis. Pulsion diverticula were considered the result of increased pressure within the lumen of the esophagus, possibly associated with motility disorders. It is now generally accepted that most if not all esophageal diverticula result from motility disturbance. One remarkable form of motility disturbance in the esophagus is achalasia, which is discussed in detail in a following section. Multiple diverticula may be seen in the presence of achalasia as well as other structural abnormalities of the esophagus, such as strictures. It has long been endoscopic lore that it is dangerous to perform esophageal dilation in the presence of diverticula, but few data support this contention. Certainly, blind dilation using mercury bougies can result in perforation of a diverticulum. Similarly, a guidewire passed without adequate precautions might do the same. These days, when tight esophageal strictures are treated, the dilators are almost always inserted over a guidewire under fluoroscopic control. These precautions afford a great deal of protection to adjacent diverticula, which should not be considered an absolute or even relative contraindication to the procedure unless there are other anatomic problems.

Figure 1-6 illustrates two hypothetical cases of multiple esophageal diverticula. In an esophagus with numerous diverticula (Figure 1-6A), the approach to the stricture is a relatively straight shot. Gentle Savary-type dilation over a guidewire under fluoroscopy should be relatively safe in this situation. Figure 1-6B represents a danger zone for the endoscopist: this esophagus has become severely tortuous, probably the result of

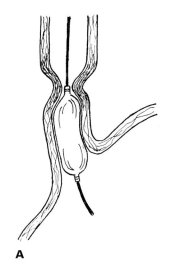

A

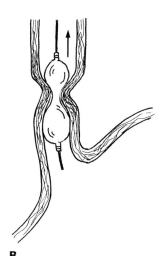

B

Figure 1-5. Self-dilation using a balloon catheter. A. The balloon dilator is advanced beyond the stricture and inflated. B. Withdrawing the inflated balloon slowly results in stricture dilation.

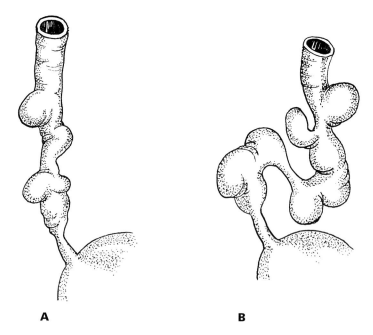

Figure 1-6. Examples of multiple esophageal diverticula. A. An esophagus with multiple diverticula where the approach is a relatively straight shot. B. An esophagus that has become severely tortuous as the result of chronic inflammatory changes. The considerable axial and radial forces generated in the process of dilating a stricture in this esophagus creates a real danger of perforation.

A   **B**

chronic inflammatory changes related to the many diverticula. The distal esophageal stricture is anything but a straight shot; considerable axial and radial forces would be generated in the process of attempting to dilate this stricture, even supposing that a flexible plastic dilator could be coaxed around all the twists and turns. Fortunately, this problem is unusual, but every endoscopist should recognize this as a high-risk situation. Surgical repair or even retrograde dilation through a gastrostomy incision may be preferable to the risk of attempted endoscopy and subsequent endoscopic dilation. When dilating an esophageal stricture associated with proximal diverticula, great care should be taken to identify the lumen positively before attempting to gently pass the guidewire. This can be considerably more difficult than it sounds due to distortion of local anatomy.

Rigid Versus Balloon Dilators

A variety of dilating balloons are available for dilating strictures in the GI tract. How do these compare with tapered plastic dilators and conventional weighted bougies? Through-the-scope (TTS) dilators have become very popular. These cylindrical or sausage-shaped plastic balloons are small enough when deflated to pass through the instrument channel of an endoscope (Figure 1-7). They can be inflated with air or fluid, the fluid often being a contrast medium, which greatly enhances the visibility of the balloon on fluoroscopy. During stricture dilation, the endoscopist can observe the balloon directly, which is a further aid to appropriate positioning. When the stricture is dilated under direct vision, it is possible to see through the balloon and watch the process take place. Although some think that direct vision increases the safety of the procedure, in reality it often just affords the endoscopist an opportunity to watch a tear or perforation occur. Plastic dilating balloons generate considerable radial forces, which may increase the risk of a perforation when dilating a tight stricture. To address this concern, dilating balloons have been designed that do not expand beyond a predetermined limit, thus limiting the radial forces.

Many endoscopists believe, however, that they have more control over the process of dilation when they pass a tapered dilator. The most common method employs a Savary-type dilator over a guidewire. With experience, one acquires a feel for the resistance generated by the stricture when the dilator is being passed. There is a knack to knowing how much pressure can be applied to overcome this resistance. My opinion is that Savary-type dilators are, indeed, safer and more predictable to use in accessible strictures of the upper GI tract. A recent prospective, randomized comparison between polyvinyl bougies and TTS balloons showed no difference in size of lumen achieved and duration of effect. TTS dilators are really the only option when dilating the pylorus or more distal duodenal strictures or webs. A distal esophageal ring (Schatzki's ring) may be more effectively dilated by a balloon with its greater radial forces than by a tapered dilator.

If there is any suspicion after dilation that a perforation has occurred, the patient should take nothing by mouth and be sent immediately for a contrast radiographic study to look for extravasation.

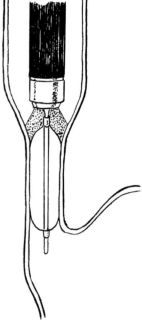

Figure 1-7. Through-the-scope balloon dilator. The process of stricture dilation is monitored under direct vision using an endoscope.

Achalasia

In achalasia of the esophagus, congenital absence of the ganglion cells of the myenteric plexus of the lower esophageal sphincter (LES) results in the sphincter being unable to relax. In long-standing cases, the esophagus progressively dilates to accommodate the solids and liquids that have difficulty passing. The contrast radiographic appearance is often highly suggestive, if not diagnostic (Figure 1-8): The gastroesophageal junction is narrow (often described as a rat tail or bird's beak) with gross proximal dilatation. In particularly marked cases, a contrast study shows chronic retention of food debris in the esophagus. Esophageal manometry showing failure of the lower sphincter to relax and disordered peristalsis in the body of the esophagus confirms the diagnosis; this should always be done before attempting endoscopic therapy, with its attendant risks. In gross cases, the diagnosis is rarely in doubt. Diagnostic difficulty may arise, however, when the lesion has not yet resulted in dilation of the esophagus above the LES. In these circumstances, the diagnosis of achalasia may be missed if it is not

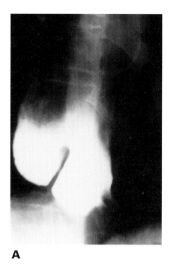
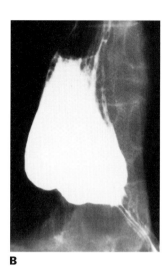

Figure 1-8. Achalasia of the esophagus in a contrast study (A) with diverticulum and (B) without diverticulum.

A   B

considered. In the past, some patients were labeled as psychiatrically disturbed for years before the true diagnosis came to light. It is an inconstant but nonetheless significant feature of the history that dysphagia is often worse for liquids than solids.

There is considerable debate about the appropriate management of achalasia. Given the risk of perforation from pneumatic dilation of achalasia and the need for repeated treatments in a significant proportion of patients, some surgeons argue that endoscopic therapy is merely a distraction on the way to a definitive surgical procedure (Heller's myotomy). Risk-benefit analysis suggests that endoscopic therapy probably has the edge and that one or two pneumatic dilations are justifiable before proceeding to surgery. The aim of pneumatic dilation is to disrupt the muscle fibers of the LES so that it becomes incompetent, thereby allowing esophageal contents to pass into the stomach. Obviously, the risk is that the forces applied will not only rupture the muscle fibers but tear the full thickness of the esophageal wall, resulting in a free perforation. Formerly, pneumatic dilation was performed using a Brown-McHardy bag, a large rubber dilating balloon on the end of a metal introducer. This balloon was positioned across the gastroesophageal junction under fluoroscopic control and inflated to achieve a pressure of about 300 mm Hg. The balloon was inflated for approximately 30 seconds, and the procedure was repeated two or three times. Because the procedure could not be performed under direct vision, the endoscopist had very little control.

Brown-McHardy dilators are no longer available. Microvasive Rigiflex pneumatic achalasia dilators (Boston Scientific Co., Watertown, MA) are in wide use and are available in three sizes: 30, 35, and 40 mm. These dilators are advanced over a Savary guidewire for accurate positioning across

the LES. Under fluoroscopic control, the midpoint of the balloon, indicated by a double radiopaque band, is positioned across the LES. When the
balloon is inflated, a waist is seen if the balloon is correctly positioned. The
waist appears at about 2 pounds per square inch (psi) and is obliterated at
about 7–9 psi, the higher pressure being maintained for 60–90 seconds.
The process should be monitored continuously because the balloon may
tend to migrate proximally when inflated. At the end of the procedure, all
air should be aspirated from the balloon before removal. Blood staining of
the balloon is thought to be a sign of an effective achalasia dilation. One
to 2 hours after the procedure, a water-soluble contrast study (esophagram)
should be performed to look for perforation, which usually occurs on the
left side of the LES. The risk of perforation is usually cited as 2–3%. If no
perforation is seen, the patient is allowed to progress to a clear liquid diet.
If no problems occur by the following morning, a normal diet may be
resumed. Unfortunately, not all perforations are immediately apparent on
an early contrast study, so a high index of suspicion for this complication
should be retained. Signs and symptoms suspicious for perforation include
persistent chest pain, pleurisy, and tachycardia.

An interesting variant of the TTS balloon (indeed, its immediate pre-
decessor) is the over-the-scope balloon (Figure 1-9). The balloon is
mounted on a sleeve that fits snugly over the shaft of the gastroscope.
With the sleeve of the balloon advanced 6 inches or so proximal to the
tip of the endoscope, a dilation at the gastroesophageal junction can be
performed under direct vision with the endoscope retroflexed. Some
believe that this technique allows better control of the dilation and direct
visualization of the results. Although over-the-scope balloons may be
available in some endoscopy units, TTS balloons have rendered their use
increasingly obsolete.

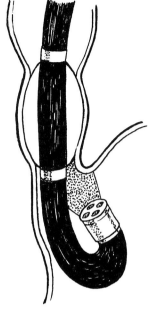

Figure 1-9. An over-the-
scope dilating balloon. The
inflated balloon at the gastroesophageal junction can
be monitored by a
retroflexed endoscope.

Botulinum Toxin

Recently, injection of botulinum toxin (Bo-Tox) into the LES has been
shown to provide transient symptomatic benefit in patients with achalasia. This is done using a sclerotherapy needle; the LES is injected in four
quadrants. The exact mechanism of action is uncertain, but it appears to
be associated with reversible destruction of acetylcholine receptors in
postganglionic neurons. Pasricha et al. randomized 21 patients with
manometrically proven achalasia to receive 80 units of botulinum toxin
or placebo. The toxin-treated patients had significantly improved dysphagia scores, reduction in LES pressure, and widening of the esophageal
lumen at the gastroesophageal junction. The treatment is relatively inex-
pensive ($300 for a vial of botulinum toxin) and free of complications,
but it does not appear to offer a long-term cure. Laparoscopic Heller's
myotomy appears to be the surgery of choice now for the definitive treatment of achalasia.

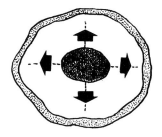

Distal Esophageal Rings

A distal esophageal (Schatzki's) ring may be an incidental finding, but it is sometimes discovered during the investigation of dysphagia or foreign body impaction. Often, these rings are subtle, but from time to time they may take up a significant proportion of the lumen of the esophagus, leaving only a small central opening. They are generally found within a few centimeters of the gastroesophageal junction. The rings are rather fibrous and often fail to respond to standard Savary-type dilation. For this reason, some endoscopists prefer to disrupt them using balloon dilators, with their ability to apply significant radial force. A number of investigators have published their experience of incising these rings using electrocautery. The idea is to make cuts in four quadrants (Figure 1-10). This can be done with an ERCP sphincterotome or a needle knife (basically a bare wire exposed at the end of a plastic catheter). Although successes have been reported, it is fair to say that this is a high-risk technique due to the potential for perforation. It should be attempted by experts only.

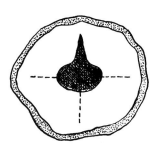

Barrett's Esophagus

Barrett's esophagus is the term given to the presence of specialized columnar epithelium in the esophagus. Specialized columnar epithelium resembles intestinal epithelium, containing both columnar and goblet cells and crypts of the type found in the small intestine. When first described by a British surgeon (N.R. Barrett) in 1950, this abnormality was believed to represent a congenital short esophagus with an intrathoracic stomach. Most experts now accept that Barrett's esophagus is an acquired condition that complicates chronic gastroesophageal reflux disease (GERD). Columnar epithelium is thought to replace squamous mucosa of the esophagus that has been damaged by acid regurgitation. Barrett's epithelium is susceptible to ulceration and stricture formation and predisposes to adenocarcinoma of the esophagus.

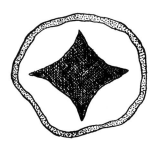

Figure 1-10. A Schatzki's ring that has resisted standard methods of dilation is opened using needle knife diathermy incisions in a four-quadrant pattern.

Screening in Barrett's Esophagus

The presence of Barrett's epithelium cannot reliably be predicted from a history of clinically significant GERD. Indeed, if the presence of columnar epithelium partially protects the esophagus from acid irritation, patients with Barrett's esophagus may be relatively less symptomatic or asymptomatic when compared with non-Barrett's patients. Given that the prevalence of Barrett's epithelium increases with age, it has been suggested that all patients aged 40 years or older with GERD of 5 years' or more duration should undergo screening endoscopy. As yet, however, there are no data to show that this strategy is cost effective.

Screening Objectives

It is often difficult to identify reliably the squamocolumnar junction between the esophagus and stomach. For this reason, it has been suggested that Barrett's esophagus exists whenever columnar epithelium is found at a distance of 3 cm or more into the tubular esophagus, recognized endoscopically as beginning where the gastric mucosal folds end. Islands of Barrett epithelium are often recognized by their pink or reddish coloration against the paler background of normal squamous mucosa of the esophagus. Endoscopic biopsies should be taken to confirm the diagnosis and to look for dysplastic changes. This should be done after the patient has been treated with a proton pump inhibitor to suppress gastric acid production. Four-quadrant biopsies should be taken every 2 cm along the affected segment.

Unfortunately, there are insufficient data on which to base recommendations for periodic screening endoscopy in Barrett's esophagus. Although we might expect that control of acid reflux by medical or surgical means would reduce the cancer risk in Barrett's esophagus, this may not be the case. Until better data regarding risk become available from long-term studies, screening in Barrett's esophagus is individualized, based on symptoms and the presence or absence of dysplasia. Clearly, this practice will miss asymptomatic patients with dysplasia or early cancer. Cost concerns in the managed care era are likely to restrict the use of endoscopy for screening, unless markers for high risk can be identified. Cytology, flow cytometry, and tumor markers, such as the p53 gene, are currently being evaluated.

Treatment for Dysplasia in Barrett's Esophagus

Many experts consider the finding of severe dysplasia in Barrett's epithelium as equivalent to carcinoma in situ. Until recently, partial or total esophagectomy has been the only treatment thought to offer a cure. Because esophagectomy is a major operation with significant long-term morbidity, endoscopic techniques are being developed to remove the abnormal epithelium. These include strip resection (mucosectomy) and photodynamic therapy using laser. Outcome data from studies of patients receiving local therapy are awaited with great interest.

Plastic Esophageal Prostheses

One of the most terrible diseases encountered by gastroenterologists is carcinoma of the esophagus, which results in progressive difficulty in swallowing (dysphagia). When the esophageal lumen becomes completely occluded by the tumor mass, the patient is unable to swallow secretions, with the inevitable result that these are aspirated into the lungs. In the past, these patients suffered a miserable death, usually due to aspiration pneumonia. Malignant tumors arising from squamous epithelium (squamous carcinomas) are generally sensitive to radiation and chemotherapy. Aggressive multiple-modality therapy for such cancers is often effective in restoring luminal patency, which allows the patient to swallow at least his or her own secretions. Malignant tumors arising in the cardia of the stomach or in heterotopic intestinal epithelium in the distal esophagus (Barrett's esophagus) are usually adenocarcinomas. These have a terrible prognosis, being almost completely insensitive to radiotherapy and chemotherapy.

In both histologic types of cancer involving the esophagus, endoscopists have a role to play in restoring and maintaining patency of the lumen. As previously discussed, standard esophageal dilation with plastic dilators or dilating balloons rarely has more than a transient effect on dysphagia. This is because the tumors tend to spring back into their original position after dilation. Mechanical efforts to widen the lumen of the occluded esophagus take two forms: the lumen can be held open artificially by a rigid prosthesis, or a variety of mainly thermal methods (e.g., laser) can be used to destroy malignant tissue and thereby recanalize the lumen. Laser and other methods of thermal ablation are discussed in the section on Ablation of Obstructing Esophageal Tumors.

Esophageal prosthesis design is rapidly evolving from reinforced plastic to coated, expandable metal mesh. Although it is certain that plastic prostheses will eventually become obsolete, they are still widely used for two reasons: (1) expandable metal mesh stent technology remains in evolution, and (2) plastic prostheses are much cheaper than metal ones. Modern esophageal prostheses have evolved into a fairly uniform design (Figure 1-11): A cylindrical body of firm plastic (usually polyethylene) is reinforced with a metal spiral. At the upper (proximal) end is a gently tapered flange and at the lower (distal) end, a longer tapering tip. These prostheses come in a variety of diameters and lengths to accommodate the varying types of malignant stricture. To place one of these prostheses, the stricture must be dilated to at least the external diameter of the device, otherwise it will not advance. Prior dilation to the desired diameter with Savary-type dilators is an essential preliminary to esophageal prosthesis (stent) placement. For the standard adult size of esophageal prosthesis, the esophagus must be able to dilate up to at least 14 mm (42 Fr). Therein lies one of the particular problems of this technique: because many esophageal tumors are extremely firm, it is possible to split the esophagus by endoscopic dilation and cause a perforation. If the tumor is associated with a large mediastinal mass, there may be tracheal compression, which can be greatly worsened by the placement of an esophageal prosthesis. A computed tomographic scan of the chest to assess the patency of the upper airway is a wise precaution before proceeding with esophageal prosthesis insertion.

The currently accepted means of inserting an esophageal prosthesis is over a plastic (Savary) dilator, which is lubricated with water-soluble gel for ease of disengagement. The prosthesis–Savary dilator combination is

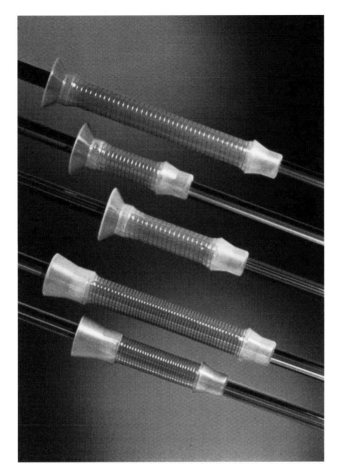

Figure 1-11. Modern plastic esophageal prostheses. (Courtesy of Wilson-Cook Medical, Inc., Winston-Salem, NC.)

advanced over a prepositioned guidewire using a plastic pusher tube to apply axial force to wedge the stent in position (Figure 1-12). This is an unpleasant procedure for both the patient and the endoscopist. Effective conscious sedation is essential. Although performing the procedure under general anesthesia might be kinder, the presence of an endotracheal tube with an inflated cuff in the upper airway sometimes provides sufficient resistance in the mediastinum to prevent a successful procedure. It is essential to know the length of the stricture so that a long enough prosthesis is chosen for the purpose. High, short esophageal strictures present a particular problem because patients are aware of a foreign body if the upper flange is left in the upper esophageal sphincter or hypopharynx. The upper and lower margins of the stricture can be determined by reading the length of endoscope inserted (from the lips) on the insertion tube (which is marked off in 5-cm intervals). A good contrast esophagram can be used for

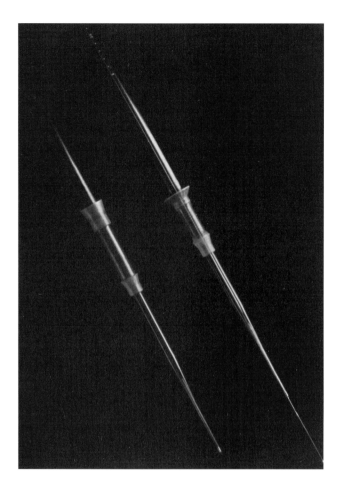

Figure 1-12. Combination prosthesis and Savary dilator advanced over a guidewire into position.

the same purpose, with the proviso of compensating for any known magnification factor. Recently, intramucosal injection of barium solution has been used as a crude but effective means of identifying the top and bottom of the stricture on fluoroscopy and plain chest radiography.

Great care must be taken to ensure that the prosthesis is advanced completely through the stricture. It is a common error to rely too heavily on predetermined measurements, which can lead to stretching of the tumor and mediastinum when axial force is applied. The entire procedure must be monitored under fluoroscopy. When the prosthesis appears to be in the desired position, the lubricated Savary dilator is removed by gently rotating it (to release the seal), then withdrawing it through the pusher tube. Once the dilator has been removed, a standard adult gastroscope (external diameter, 11 mm) can be advanced through the pusher tube to inspect the position of the prosthesis. If this is found to be inadequate (usually not far enough in), the dilator can be repositioned and further pressure applied from above to advance the prosthesis. Throughout the procedure, the endoscopist must be alert to the possibility of airway obstruction. An inadequately sedated patient will struggle, often violently, during insertion of what is a large foreign body through the upper esophageal sphincter. If this occurs, or if there is obvious stridor (noisy, obstructed respiration), the pusher tube should be removed immediately and the prosthesis grasped by the endoscopist's thumb and forefinger inserted through the mouth. Provided that the upper flange of the tube has not already crossed the upper esophageal sphincter, it can usually be withdrawn without difficulty.

Sometimes, the stent passes into the esophagus but fails to traverse the stricture. In this position, it is obviously beyond the reach of fingers. The maker of the standard esophageal prosthesis provides a retrieval balloon that can be inflated within the lumen of the stent to allow it to be withdrawn. From personal experience, I consider this an indispensable part of the equipment needed to safely perform esophageal stent placement. Although it may seem logical to attempt to snare the flange of the stent to facilitate withdrawal, this is often less than satisfactory because the stent inevitably ends up being pulled at an angle, with a high risk of trauma to the upper esophageal sphincter. If the esophageal stent has advanced too far, it is possible to use the retrieval device for repositioning. The balloon is inflated within the stent, which is pulled back into the desired position. In the unusual circumstance of a stent ending up way beyond its desired position, an alternative means of retrieval is to push the stent into the stomach, then snare it by the lower (distal) end. The stent can then be pulled up through the esophagus by its narrow end. This procedure is traumatic—for both the patient and the endoscopist—and efforts should be made to avoid the need for it.

Tracheoesophageal Fistula

A modification of the esophageal prosthesis is used to manage the difficult problem of a tracheoesophageal or bronchoesophageal fistula (Figure 1-13A). This commonly results from irradiation of esophageal or lung cancer. The fistulous connection between the esophagus and the respiratory tree has a classic presentation: The patient coughs whenever he or she eats or drinks. In the past, there was no satisfactory solution for this problem, but a recent modification of a commercially available esophageal stent has an expandable foam-filled cuff whose purpose is to occlude the fistula (Figure 1-14). This ingenious device can provide effective palliation for patients with exophytic tumors in the esophagus associated with fistulae to the respiratory tree. The stent is inserted with the foam-filled cuff deflated (Figure 1-13B). This is achieved by applying suction (using a syringe) through a detachable thin plastic tube. Once the prosthesis is in the desired position, the side tube is detached by a sharp tug while the stent is held in

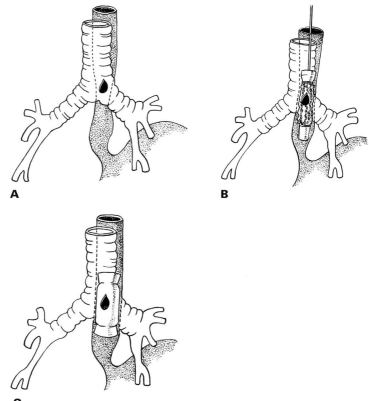

Figure 1-13. A. Tracheo-esophageal fistula. B. Cuffed esophageal stent inserted with cuff deflated. C. Occlusion of the fistula by the inflated foam-filled cuff.

position with a pusher tube. A small hole left at the tube insertion site allows air to expand the foam-filled sleeve. The result is occlusion of the fistula by the sleeve (Figure 1-13C). It should be emphasized that this technique can only be used when there is sufficient tumor mass to hold the inflated stent in place. This means that the tumor either needs to be exophytic or that there is sufficient extrinsic compression to hold the tube in place.

I am sometimes asked to consider stenting for tracheoesophageal or bronchoesophageal fistulae in patients who have received irradiation for endobronchial tumors. Because these patients generally have no mass involving the esophagus, it is unsafe to leave an esophageal stent with an expandable cuff for palliation. Unless the stent is anchored in a suitable position, it may migrate proximally in the middle of the night and choke the patient. It has recently been suggested that a modification of the foam cuff stent could be used to apply chemotherapy directly to the surface of the tumor, thereby enhancing the drugs' effect. This is an intriguing possibility but one that remains to be tested in clinical trials. Cuffed plastic pros-

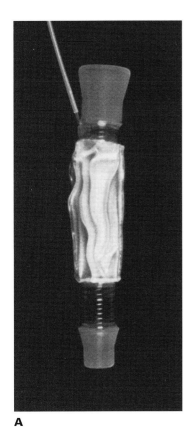 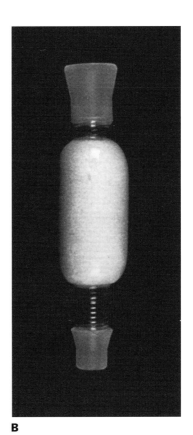

A   B

Figure 1-14. Uninflated (A) and inflated (B) esophageal prosthesis with foam-filled cuff. Such prostheses are used to occlude respiratory-esophageal fistula. (Courtesy of Wilson-Cook Medical, Inc., Winston-Salem, NC.)

theses are likely to become obsolete soon with the development of coated metal mesh stents for use in the esophagus.

Metal Mesh Stents

A promising technology is that of expandable metallic mesh stents for esophageal use (Figure 1-15). Expandable metal stents have been used for some time in malignant bile duct obstruction, but they can also be used in the esophagus for a similar purpose, namely, holding open malignant strictures. A major limitation of the original metal mesh stents was the tendency for tumor to grow through the interstices, causing late occlusion. Several metallic mesh stents with flexible plastic covers are now being marketed in the United States for use in the esophagus. It is anticipated that covered metal stents will have a significant role in palliating tracheoesophageal and bronchoesophageal fistulae.

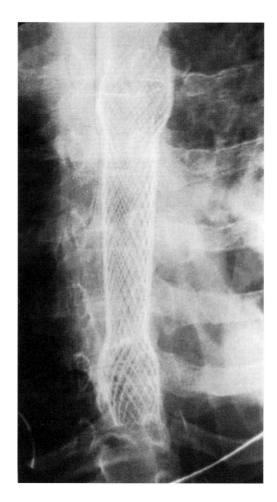

Figure 1-15. Expandable metal mesh stent in esophagus.

A major advantage of metal mesh stents in the esophagus is the ability to place them through a relatively small lumen. At present, expandable mesh stents for use in the biliary tree are only 8 Fr (< 3 mm) in external diameter in their undeployed state. Metallic mesh stents for use in the esophagus will require similar delivery systems. This reduces the requirement to dilate the lumen of the tumor greatly before a prosthesis can be placed, which causes many of the complications of this procedure. It will certainly make it a less uncomfortable procedure for the patient. The metallic stent requires room to expand, however. If the lumen is narrow and the tumor inelastic, the stent may fail to deploy to its maximum diameter. At present, a limitation of expandable metal mesh stents is their permanence: once deployed, they are difficult to remove (Figure 1-16).

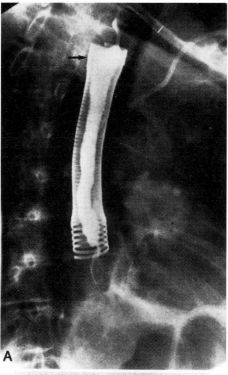

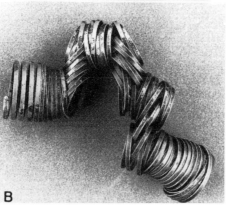

Figure 1-16. A. A nitinol stent in position in the esophagus. Once deployed, they are difficult to remove. B. The remains of a nitinol stent after endoscopic removal.

Another problem is that some metal stents tend to migrate distally despite their large external diameter. This is a particular problem when patients receive chemotherapy or irradiation with the stent in place. If the tumor responds by shrinking, the stent is likely to migrate. To discourage migration, tiny hooks are added to some metal stents to encourage them to maintain position. A new generation of metallic stents made from "memo-

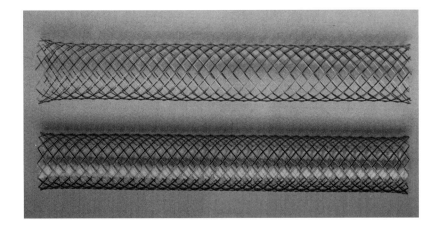

Figure 1-17. Uncoated (top) and coated (bottom) metal mesh stents. (Courtesy of Schneider [USA], Minneapolis, MN.)

ry metals" should facilitate their removal because some of these metals become soft and elastic when cooled with ice water. The new generation of metal mesh stents have plastic coatings to prevent tumor ingrowth (Figure 1-17). They are slippery and therefore easier to remove or reposition, but they are also more prone to migration. Uncoated metal mesh stents have a tendency to occlude due to tumor ingrowth. Photodynamic therapy has been used recently to destroy tumor growing through the interstices of an uncoated metallic esophageal stent.

Kozarek et al. have reported that patients with esophageal cancer do equally poorly regardless of the type of prosthesis they receive. Conventional (plastic) and metal mesh stents are both associated with significant complications. As Fleischer points out in an accompanying editorial, however, metal stents are undoubtedly easier to place, which reduces the discomfort and morbidity of the procedure. As metal mesh stents are much more expensive than plastic ones, cost-benefit studies are eagerly awaited. Several experts in the field have recommended that endoscopists retain a selection of conventional (plastic) esophageal stents in their inventory of accessories, at least until more data are available regarding the benefits and risks of metal stents.

Ablation of Obstructing Esophageal Tumors

Thermal Methods

A variety of techniques have been developed to destroy cancerous tissue obstructing the esophagus, with the aim of restoring luminal patency. Thermal ablation using the neodymium-yttrium-aluminum-garnet (Nd:YAG) laser to vaporize tissue is probably the most widely used for this purpose. If the malignant stricture is tight, and the endoscope cannot easily be advanced beyond it, even after dilatation, laser treatment is applied in concentric rings around what remains of the lumen. If the stricture can be crossed, the endoscopist may choose to treat the distal end of the tumor first, working upward. This is thought to provide more control of the photocoagulation process. Power settings of 50–100 W and pulse durations of 1 second or more are usually required to coagulate and vaporize malignant tissue. Tumor ablation by laser often requires multiple treatment sessions: Several days after each treatment, necrotic tissue is removed and additional laser energy is applied to the remaining tumor. Contact lasers do not appear to offer any benefit over noncontact lasers in this situation. Photodynamic therapy to enhance the action of laser tumor ablation remains experimental at this time (see Chapter 4, section on Lasers in Endoscopy). With skill and care, a useful lumen can be restored to allow the patient to swallow. Unfortunately, restoration of luminal patency rarely results in normal swallowing: The patient may have persistent dysphagia (usually worse for solids) due to loss of normal esophageal peristalsis. However, most patients undergoing laser therapy have advanced disease and may have little desire to eat. The ability to swallow secretions and maintain hydration orally is usually regarded as successful palliation for malignant dysphagia. As one would expect, applying thermal energy in this way is not without risk, with perforation and bleeding as recognized complications. Although mild fever may follow laser photocoagulation therapy, high fever, persistent fever beyond 24 hours, or chest pain should raise suspicion of iatrogenic perforation. A water-soluble contrast (e.g., Gastrograffin [Bracco Diagnostics, Princeton, NJ]) study of the esophagus should be performed to assess the problem.

Another way to apply thermal energy is to use a Bicap probe. This device applies heat energy in a radial fashion. Multiple, parallel electrodes on an olive-shaped dilator allow the application of bipolar electrocoagulation as the probe is pushed through the malignant stricture (over a guidewire). Probes are available in diameters of 6–15 mm. They can be used under direct vision (Figure 1-18), i.e., monitoring probe position by endoscopy, or with fluoroscopy, especially when treatment is applied in a retrograde fashion, i.e., from the bottom of the stricture upward (Figure 1-19). Although the Bicap probe has been used successfully by numerous investigators, it has failed to gain widespread acceptance, possibly because it is perceived to offer less control than laser does over site and depth of thermal injury. The Bicap probe should not be used for noncircumferential tumors. Delayed bleeding, tracheoesophageal fistulae, and late strictures have all been reported with this technique. A tumor probe employing microwave radiation has also been evaluated and appears to offer similar results.

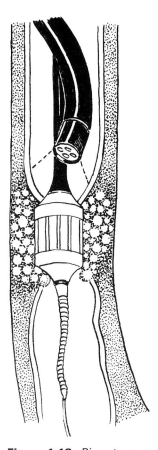

Figure 1-18. Bicap tumor probe being used under direct vision.

Chemical Necrolysis

A "cheap and cheerful" alternative to thermal ablation of obstructing tumors is chemically induced necrosis by injection of polidocanol or

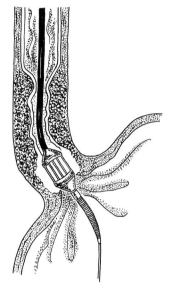

Figure 1-19. Bicap tumor probe applied in a retrograde fashion.

absolute alcohol: 0.5- to 1.0-ml aliquots are injected deeply into the tumor at multiple sites. The results are best for firm, bulky tumors and poorest for friable tumors.

Brachytherapy and External Beam Irradiation

Brachytherapy (local irradiation) using iridium 192 or cesium 137 sources positioned within the tumor lumen (using a remote loading device) has been shown to shrink esophageal tumors but at the expense of significant radiation esophagitis. One (uncontrolled) study of external beam radiotherapy suggested that the administration of a 15- to 30-Gy dose of radiation after laser photocoagulation may almost double the dysphagia-free interval in patients with squamous carcinoma.

Endoscopic Treatment of Nonvariceal Upper Gastrointestinal Hemorrhage

Upper GI hemorrhage is a frequent problem requiring the intervention of endoscopists. Early diagnosis and, where appropriate, endoscopic therapy reduce the morbidity and mortality from bleeding. Table 1-1 lists the principal causes of severe upper GI hemorrhage and continuing hemorrhage in 200 conservative patients admitted to Los Angeles hospitals.

Thermal and injection techniques have been widely adopted (Table 1-2). Glue is difficult to contain and has the potential to damage the endoscope channel. In the hands of enthusiasts, mechanical devices appear to work well, but none has gained popular support.

Table 1-1. List of the principal causes of severe upper gastrointestinal hemorrhage and continuing hemorrhage in 200 consecutive patients admitted to Los Angeles hospitals

Diagnosis	Frequency (%)	Continuing bleeding (%)
Peptic ulcers	50	28
Esophageal and gastric varices	22	46
Angiodysplasia	7.5	7
Mallory-Weiss tears	6	17
Upper gastrointestinal cancers	5	10
Gastric or duodenal erosions	4.5	0
Other	4.5	11

Source: Adapted from DM Jensen. Presented at the American Society for Gastrointestinal Endoscopy Postgraduate Course, 1995.

Table 1-2. Methods to control upper gastrointestinal hemorrhage

Thermal (heater probe)
    Bipolar cautery (Bicap, Gold Probe)
    Microwave
    Laser
Injection (sclerosants)
    Epinephrine (adrenaline)
    Saline (normal or hypertonic)
    Alcohol
    Trimethylaminoethanesulfonic acid
    Sodium morrhuate
    Sodium tetradecylsulfate
Glue
    Cyanoacrylate ("super glue")
Mechanical devices (endoscopic clips)
    Banding
    "Sewing machine"
    Ferromagnetic

Source: Adapted from DM Jensen. Presented at the American Society for
Gastrointestinal Endoscopy Postgraduate Course, 1995.

Which lesions require endoscopic therapy—and with which modality—are questions that remain hotly debated. Considerable attention has been given to the stigmata of recent hemorrhage. These range from the visible vessel to the ulcer with overlying clot and the so-called flat spots. Table 1-3 shows the rebleeding rates for 140 ulcer patients with stigmata of recent hemorrhage (data combined from three studies from one center in London).

Table 1-4 shows the outcomes of 100 intensive care unit patients with severe ulcer bleeding who received medical therapy for an ulcer identified at endoscopy but no endoscopic treatment.

Randomized controlled trials of treatment by laser, Bicap probe, and epinephrine injection for active bleeding or stigmata of recent hemorrhage, or both, have shown that these endoscopic treatments provide effective immediate hemostasis, reduce the need for transfusion and emergency surgery, and reduce the cost and duration of hospitalization. The 1989 study by Laine of Bicap for nonbleeding visible vessels is typical (Table 1-5).

How Should Endoscopic Methods of Hemostasis Be Used?

The decision to use one or more of the available endoscopic therapies depends on the clinical situation and on the accessibility of the bleeding site.

Table 1-3. Rebleeding rates for 140 ulcer patients with stigmata of recent hemorrhage

Endoscopic stigmata	Prevalence (%)	More bleeding (%)
Major		
Visible vessel, bleeding	11.5	70.6
Visible vessel, nonbleeding	54.7	50.6
Minor		
Overlying clot, bleeding	7.4	36.0
Overlying clot, nonbleeding	7.4	9.0
Flat spots, bleeding	6.8	10.0
Flat spots, nonbleeding	12.2	0

Source: Adapted from DM Jensen. Presented at the American Society for Gastrointestinal Endoscopy Postgraduate Course, 1995.

Table 1-4. Outcome of 100 intensive care unit patients with severe ulcer bleeding who received medical therapy for an ulcer identified at endoscopy but no endoscopic treatment

Endoscopic appearance	Percent of total (%)	More bleeding (%)
Active bleeding	16	88
Nonbleeding visible vessel	22	50
Nonbleeding clot	15	33
Gray slough, flat red/black spot	14	7
Clean ulcer base	33	3

Source: Reprinted with permission from TOG Kovaks, M Jensen. Endoscopic control of gastroduodenal hemorrhage. Annu Rev Med 1987;38:267.

Heater probes, Bicap, and other treatment methods can be used tangentially, which give them a distinct advantage over laser, which requires a clear target. Injections can be made without clearly identifying a point bleeding source (i.e., the vicinity of the bleeding can be treated). Some experts recommend the combination of injection and thermal therapies. Injection of epinephrine, saline, or sclerosant solution often creates a bloodless field, which renders subsequent thermal ablation of the offending vessel technically straightforward. A thermal Gold Probe (Boston Scientific Corp., Watertown, MA) with a built-in injector is currently being marketed.

Thermal methods rely on coagulation of tissue and, in the case of probes, pressure effects to cause hemostasis. Pressure over a vessel during electrocoagulation will fuse, or coapt, the walls together (Figure 1-20). Thus, sufficient power must be applied for enough time and with sustained pressure to maximize the effect. Overcautious application of thermal energy gives a suboptimal result. Some experts recommend

Table 1-5. Medical therapy (control) versus Bicap probe for treatment of nonbleeding visible vessels

Treatment	Control	Bicap
Number of patients	37	38
Definitive hemostasis	18%	41%*
Red blood cell transfusions	3.0 U	1.6 U*
Emergency surgery	30%	8%*
Hospital days	6.2	4.3*
Overall cost	$5,630	$3,790
Mortality	0%	3%

*Statistically significant difference ($P < 0.05$).
Source: Adapted from DM Jensen. Presented at the American Society for Gastrointestinal Endoscopy Postgraduate Course, 1995.

pulse durations of up to 10 seconds when using thermal probes at power settings of around 30 J. These long, powerful bursts of thermal energy are repeated until active bleeding stops or visible vessels are flattened. Laine has termed this a "scorched earth" approach. Power settings and durations are reduced for Mallory-Weiss tears, Dieulafoy lesions, and angiodysplasia. Power, pressure, and duration settings must also be reduced for small, superficial, or deep bleeding lesions. Large-diameter thermal probes (approximately 3.2 mm in diameter) are recommended for all but the smallest lesions. These should be used through large-channel endoscopes (preferably double-channel) when there is active upper GI hemorrhage.

Injection therapy is usually applied through a standard sclerotherapy needle (Figure 1-21). Recent studies suggest that tissue pressure may be as important as the local pharmacologic effect. Therefore, injection of 5 ml or more of hemostatic agents in the vicinity of the bleeding vessel is not inappropriate. The pressure of fluid in the tissues is thought to compress local arteries, with reduction in flow. Sclerosants and epinephrine cause smooth muscle spasm, further reducing arterial flow. Absolute alcohol and trimethylaminoethanesulfonic acid (TES) dehydrate and thus locally "fix" tissue, but they also predispose to tissue necrosis and ulceration.

Laser therapy is limited by its expense, lack of portability, and the need for a clear, end-on target; noncontact probes cannot be used tangentially. The Nd:YAG laser is the most commonly used laser for endoscopic hemostasis. In experienced hands, endoscopic laser photocoagulation can be very effective, but care must be taken to avoid vaporizing tissue around the ulcer and its base, which may exacerbate bleeding if a feeding artery is punctured. Recently, the water-guided laser has been introduced. A jet of water not only carries the laser light but cools the surface being treated, thus limiting vaporization. When laser is being used to treat upper GI bleeding, standard laser precautions must be observed. In addition, some means of venting

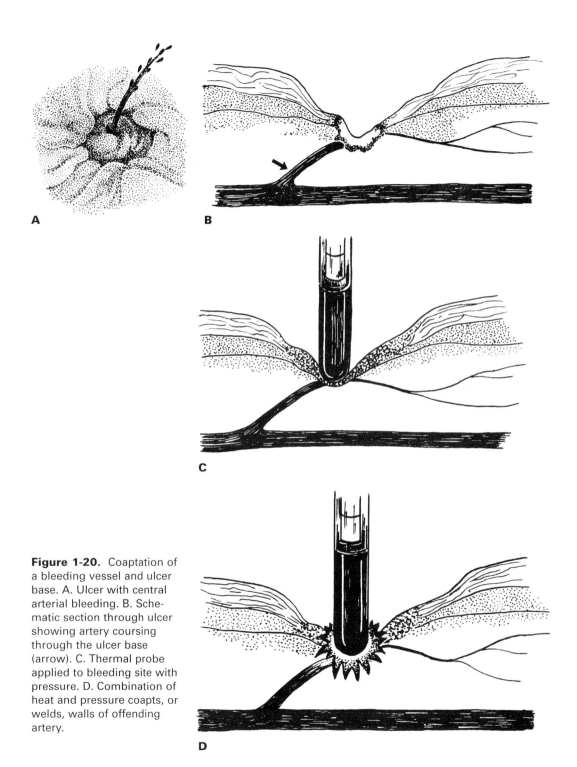

Figure 1-20. Coaptation of a bleeding vessel and ulcer base. A. Ulcer with central arterial bleeding. B. Schematic section through ulcer showing artery coursing through the ulcer base (arrow). C. Thermal probe applied to bleeding site with pressure. D. Combination of heat and pressure coapts, or welds, walls of offending artery.

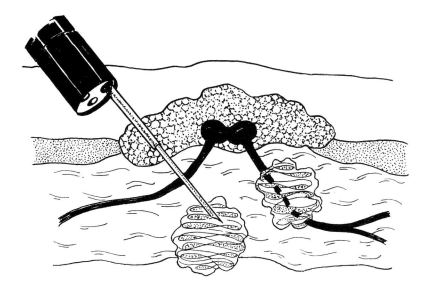

Figure 1-21. Sclerotherapy (injection) needle being used to inject an ulcer base.

coolant gas must be provided, such as a nasogastric tube; otherwise, the patient quickly becomes distended and may vomit gastric contents. As the standard laser probes are of the noncontact variety, laser photocoagulation does not allow application of pressure to the bleeding site.

Ultimately, the choice of endoscopic therapy lies with the individual operator. Price, portability, ease of use, and effectiveness are relevant to this decision. Thermal and injection methods are likely to remain the popular choices in the foreseeable future.

Esophageal and Gastric Varices

Endoscopic therapy for bleeding varices can be applied in the acute setting, while the varices are actively bleeding, or after bleeding has stopped. Patients with profuse hemorrhage from esophageal varices may be stabilized by balloon tamponade (Sengstaken or Minnesota tube) with or without prior pharmacotherapy (e.g., octreotide, vasopressin, or nitroglycerin).

Currently available endoscopic treatment options for varices include sclerosant injection, band ligation, combination sclerotherapy and band ligation, glues (including cyanoacrylate ["superglue"] and fibrin glue), and hemostatic clip ligation.

1. *Sclerosant injection* remains the most widely used technique for control of bleeding varices. Large volumes (20–30 ml) of sclerosant may need to be injected (preferably by the intravariceal route) at each treatment ses-

sion. Sclerotherapy is associated with numerous complications, including local ulceration, perforation, stricture formation, rebleeding, mediastinitis, pleural effusion, and pericarditis.

2. *Band ligation* has shown significant promise as a less morbid alternative to injection sclerotherapy. In this technique, a plastic cap attached to the end of a standard gastroscope is used to place a rubber band (O-ring) around a varix, causing it to thrombose and eventually slough off. After the target is sucked into the lumen of the banding cap (Figure 1-22A), a preloaded rubber band is ejected over the neck of the varix (Figure 1-22B), where it draws in the tissue, occluding the venous flow (Figure 1-22C). (At the end of the procedure, the O-ring is left tightly adherent to the varix, which will necrose and slough off; Figure 1-22D.) With the original device, the endoscope had to be withdrawn and reloaded after each treatment, which added considerably to the time required. Multiple-band delivery systems are now available; these have greatly reduced the time required to band multiple varices (Figure 1-23). Overall, band ligation of nonbleeding varices is easier to perform than injection sclerotherapy and is probably associated with fewer complications. In the setting of acute variceal bleeding, however, sclerotherapy may be easier to use given the lack of a clear field of view. Laine and Cook have performed a useful meta-analysis comparing the two treatment modalities.

3. *Combined variceal band ligation and sclerotherapy* has been advocated by some authors, especially for gastric varices, which have large feeding vessels. This belt-and-braces approach has appeal, but so far data are lacking regarding its efficacy.

4. *Glues*

a. *Cyanoacrylate* ("superglue") is a rapid-setting household glue. Provided that it can be used in a contained system that prevents damage to the endoscope, cyanoacrylate can be effective in controlling hemorrhage, presumably by plugging the feeding veins. The glue has to be injected into the varix; surface application is ineffective.

b. *Fibrin glue* is a biological glue made up of fibrinogen and thrombin. When these two substances combine, the result is a clot. To separate them prior to mixing, a double-channel needle injector is required. Although this type of glue is attractive because it is physiologic, provoking intravascular thrombosis in this fashion has its risks.

5. *Hemostatic clip ligation* (metallic clips) have been used to control bleeding from ulcers and polypectomy sites. The endoscopic clip ligator can place a single clip at a time. Because the currently available clips are just 7 mm wide, only small varices can be clipped effectively. Several clips may have to be applied to ensure control of bleeding. The clips slough off after several weeks. There is limited experience with this technique, but a potential complication is tearing of a varix during application, with subsequent hemorrhage.

For urgent decompression of esophageal and gastric varices, the transjugular intrahepatic portosystemic shunt (TIPS) procedure, performed by vas-

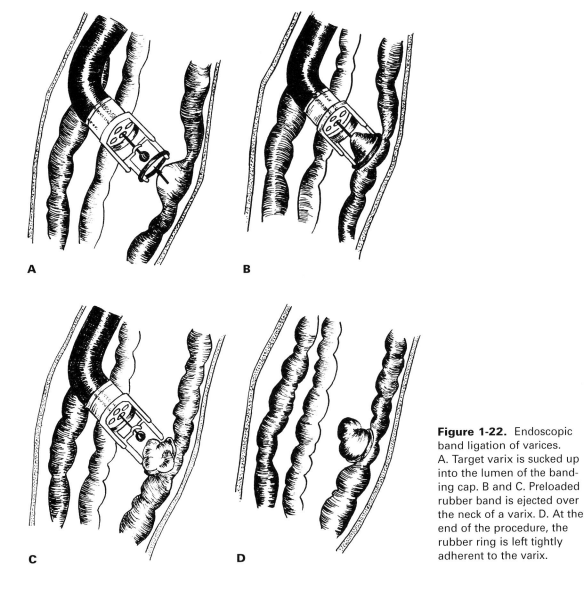

A

B

C

D

Figure 1-22. Endoscopic band ligation of varices. A. Target varix is sucked up into the lumen of the banding cap. B and C. Preloaded rubber band is ejected over the neck of a varix. D. At the end of the procedure, the rubber ring is left tightly adherent to the varix.

cular radiologists, has proved very effective. TIPS should be considered in patients who fail conventional endoscopic therapy for acutely bleeding or recurrent varices. TIPS is also beneficial in the management of resistant ascites. In the TIPS procedure, a fistula between the portal and hepatic (systemic) venous systems is established using an expandable metal mesh stent (Figure 1-24).

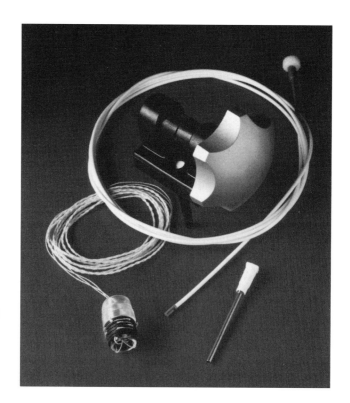

Figure 1-23. Multiple band delivery system for esophageal varix ligation. (Courtesy of Wilson-Cook Medical, Inc., Winston-Salem, NC.)

Submucosal Masses

Submucosal masses present a challenge to endoscopists because they are not readily accessible to standard techniques for biopsy and removal. The majority of submucosal masses I see are benign cystic structures, but large or enlarging masses are worrisome and require a histologic diagnosis. Submucosal masses by definition have a normal-looking surface (mucosa). Cystic masses usually have a regular, rounded appearance, and some are fluctuant when probed with catheters or forceps. Lipomas (benign tumors of fat cells) especially display this quality (the pillow sign).

Endoscopic ultrasound is useful in defining many submucosal masses. It is often possible to distinguish benign from malignant disease. A benign cyst has a well-defined structure with no evidence of invasion through or beyond it (Figure 1-25). If there is reasonable confidence that the lesion is not a vascular tumor (e.g., hemangioma), and the mass is endoscopically accessible, it is reasonable to attempt resection. An elegant way to do this is to deroof the structure, exposing the nucleus of the cyst (Figure 1-26A). If the base of the structure is then squeezed with a snare, the contents usually protrude and are sometimes expelled entirely (Figure 1-26B). If the

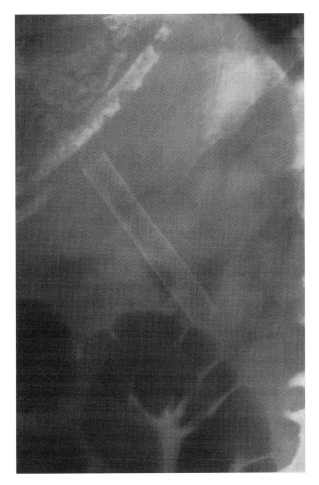

Figure 1-24. Wallstent (Schneider [USA] Inc., Minneapolis, MN) used for transjugular intrahepatic portosystemic shunt procedure.

core of the mass resists this approach, the snare can be used to resect it by electrocautery (Figure 1-26C). If it is not possible or prudent to remove the submucosal mass, repeated biopsies at the same site (tunnel biopsy technique) may reveal its contents.

Percutaneous Gastrostomy and Percutaneous Jejunostomy

Percutaneous gastrostomy (PEG) and jejunostomy (PEJ) tube placement have been available for more than 10 years now and are firmly established as safe and effective means to achieve a variety of goals. The following comments apply principally to PEG, but many are also directly applicable

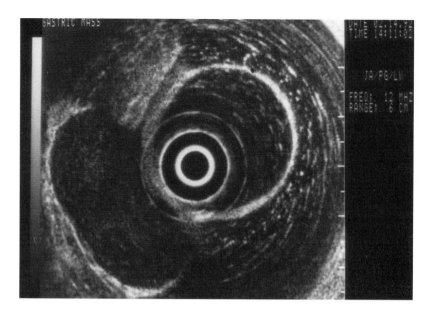

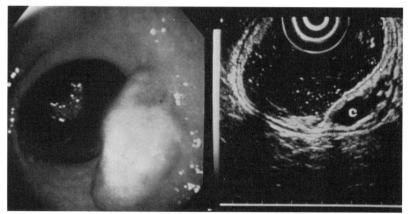

Figure 1-25. Endoscopic ultrasound image used to define benign gut wall cysts. The concentric circles seen on the image are unique to this type of imaging. The ultrasound transducer is housed within an inflatable water balloon. The center of the image (the innermost circle) corresponds to the long axis of the endoscope.

to PEJ. The list of indications for PEG placement has expanded considerably from the principal one—feeding patients with chronic, stable neurologic deficits (usually stroke) who cannot swallow. Expanded uses include the following:

- Decompression of the stomach and small bowel in carcinomatoses
- Decompression in postoperative ileus
- Management of gastric volvulus
- Access for endoscopy (including pancreatic pseudocyst decompression)

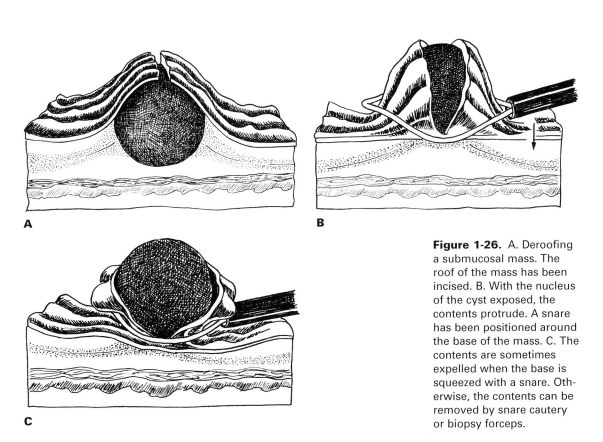

A

B

C

Figure 1-26. A. Deroofing a submucosal mass. The roof of the mass has been incised. B. With the nucleus of the cyst exposed, the contents protrude. A snare has been positioned around the base of the mass. C. The contents are sometimes expelled when the base is squeezed with a snare. Otherwise, the contents can be removed by snare cautery or biopsy forceps.

- Long-term administration of unpalatable substances, such as bile
- Retrograde esophageal dilatation and stenting

Numerous kits for PEG (and PEJ) insertion are commercially available. Despite increasingly clever solutions to the problem of placing these tubes, the basic techniques are unchanged. One method is to use a silk suture advanced through a trochar into the stomach to pull the gastrostomy tube from the mouth into the stomach and out through the abdominal wall (the pull technique). First, the most suitable site for PEG insertion into the stomach is identified by digital probing. Under direct endoscopic vision, the endoscopist or an assistant probes the upper abdomen with a finger to pinpoint a suitable puncture site (Figure 1-27A). This is monitored endoscopically to ensure that the puncture site will not coincide with visible blood vessels. The target area should be at least two fingerbreadths below the costal margin. After local anesthesia, a trochar and cannula (of the type used for venous access) are pushed through the abdominal wall into the distended stomach (Figure 1-27B). The central stylet (trochar) is removed and a silk thread, or a guidewire, is passed through the lumen of the can-

Figure 1-27. A. Percutaneous gastrostomy. The endoscopist probes the abdomen with a finger to pinpoint a suitable puncture site. B. Percutaneous gastrostomy. After local anesthesia, trocar and cannula are pushed through the abdominal wall into the stomach distended with air. C. Percutaneous gastrostomy. Wire is grasped with endoscopic snare and pulled up through the endoscope or the esophagus.

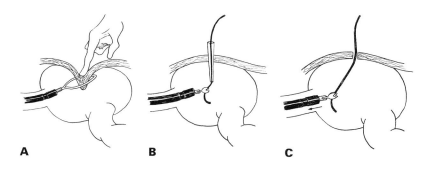

A   B   C

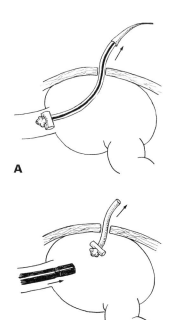

Figure 1-28. A. Percutaneous gastrostomy. The tube is delivered through the abdominal wall. B. Final positioning of percutaneous gastrostomy tube is monitored under direct vision.

nula into the stomach. In certain PEG systems, this thread or wire is grasped with an endoscopic snare and pulled up through the endoscope (Figure 1-27C).

In other methods (e.g., the BARD PEG system [CR Bard, Inc., Billerica, MA]), the wire, snare, and endoscope are removed as a unit. The wire is then threaded through the gastrostomy tube, which is then pushed or pulled through the esophagus into the stomach and out through the abdominal wall (Figure 1-28A). The final positioning of the tube is monitored under direct vision by the endoscopist (Figure 1-28B). A small scalpel incision is usually needed to enlarge the opening in the abdominal wall. It is essential to avoid an excessively tight fit, which may encourage tissue necrosis and subsequent infection. The final step is to secure the tube against the abdominal wall using a plastic bumper. The fit should be snug but not under tension. The gastrostomy tube should not be used immediately. It is usually safe to use if the patient appears comfortable and the site looks healthy after 24 hours. A small pneumoperitoneum is common after PEG placement; it resolves over 7–10 days.

A variety of compact PEG devices are now available; they are most commonly used as replacement tubes once the initial percutaneous tract has matured. One form of compact PEG has a simple button system, which is easy for patients and their attendants to use (Figures 1-29A and B). The gastrostomy orifice can be used to provide access for a jejunal feeding tube. PEJ is intended to reduce the risk of reflux and aspiration, but the results have been disappointing. Particular problems with PEJ tubes include proximal migration (into the stomach), clogging, and loss of access to the stomach for administration of drugs. Surgical (often laparoscopic) jejunostomy tube placement, which offers more distal access for feeding, is increasing in popularity as an alternative.

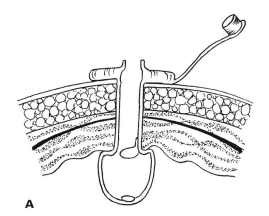 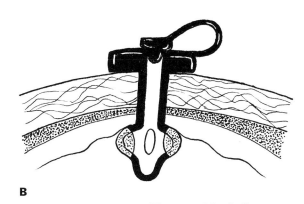

Figure 1-29. A. Compact percutaneous gastrostomy device with a simple button system. B. Button device with access port sealed.

Ingested Foreign Bodies

The ability to manage ingested foreign bodies safely and effectively is a basic skill for all GI endoscopists. An extensive discussion of foreign bodies is beyond the scope of this book. Some of the basic issues have already been discussed in a companion textbook (J Baillie. Gastrointestinal Endoscopy: Basic Principles and Practice. Oxford, England: Butterworth–Heinemann, 1992). The most common type of foreign body seen by the adult gastroenterologist is probably meat impacted above a stricture or ring in the esophagus. When the gastroenterologist is called to help manage a patient with dysphagia related to meat bolus impaction, it is important to establish the severity of the dysphagia and the duration of the problem, both of which influence management.

A patient who cannot swallow saliva represents a medical emergency and requires urgent attention. A patient who has a sensation of retrosternal sticking but can get fluids (including saliva) down the esophagus is in less danger but nonetheless requires an active treatment plan. If the meat (often chicken) has been impacted for only a few hours, it will be fairly solid, which makes it relatively easy to entrap in a basket catheter, snare, or the tip of an endoscopic overtube. Wedging a meat bolus into the tip of an endoscopic overtube and then retracting the tube can be an effective way to remove this common foreign body. After the first few hours, digestion by salivary enzymes renders the meat increasingly soft and difficult to manipulate. When meat has turned to mush, it may be possible to push it through the stricture or ring by gentle pressure with open biopsy forceps. Sometimes the simple act of insufflating through the endoscope blows the offending meat bolus through a web or stricture into the stomach. When the meat bolus has been present for many hours, there is usually an inflammatory response in a ring around the foreign body. When this occurs in the

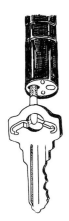

Figure 1-30. Ingested foreign body. Cups of a forceps hold a key in place as it is withdrawn.

vicinity of a stricture or a web, caution must be exercised in dilating the narrow area. Some endoscopists choose to delay formal stricture dilation until such inflammatory reactions have had time to resolve.

Patients with meat bolus impaction should never be given meat tenderizer to drink. This fluid contains papain, a proteolytic enzyme. Although it may be administered with good intentions, the result is often an intense inflammatory response, and cases of esophageal perforation have been reported. Patients with a history of meat bolus impaction should be educated about the foods most likely to give them trouble. I ask patients to remember their ABCs: *A* stands for apple (a reminder about fibrous fruits), *B* stands for bread (unchewed bread is a common culprit), and *C* stands for chicken (a reminder about fibrous meats). These patients should also be instructed to keep carbonated drinks in the refrigerator. The agitation caused by the bubbles released from these drinks may help dislodge transiently obstructing food boluses.

Certain types of foreign body are difficult to deal with. Some ingenious techniques have been devised to retrieve them safely. Keys may be left to pass spontaneously through the GI tract in adults, depending on their size, but a large door key may fail to advance in a baby or toddler and would have to be retrieved. A key with a hole in the head can be grasped by passing the tip of a biopsy forceps through the hole and opening the forceps. The cups of the forceps hold the key in place as it is withdrawn (Figure 1-30).

A safety pin requires particular care due to the sharp tip. It has been known for many years that a safety pin pulled out with the sharp tip trailing is far less likely to cause a perforation than if it is withdrawn with the tip pointing forward. If a safety pin in the esophagus can be safely coaxed into the stomach, this is a far safer place to attempt retrieval maneuvers. If a snare can be advanced over the open safety pin, closure can result in the pin locking shut, which renders the object harmless (Figure 1-31). This is

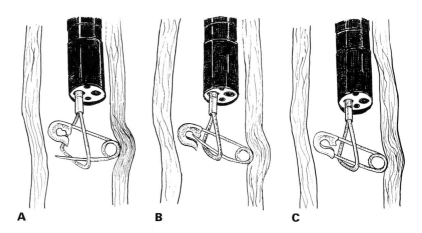

Figure 1-31. Ingested foreign body. (A) A safety pin is trapped with a snare, (B) closed with the snare, and (C) ready to be withdrawn.

A   **B**   **C**

more easily said than done, however. If the safety pin cannot be closed using the technique described, consider pulling the open pin against the tip of the scope, where the sharp point of the pin can be trapped (Figure 1-32). With the safety pin held in this position, it can be safely withdrawn. Consideration should be given to performing these maneuvers through an endoscopic overtube, which provides important protection for the upper airway. It is not helpful to retrieve a safety pin from the stomach or esophagus only to have it aspirated into the patient's upper airway.

The endoscopic overtube itself may be used to entrap certain foreign bodies, such as an impacted meat bolus. The overtube is advanced with the endoscope down to the level of the impaction, and vigorous suction is applied (Figure 1-33A). This may result in the offending object being sucked into the end of the overtube, with which it can be withdrawn (Figure 1-33B).

A flexible rubber cup that slips over the end of the endoscope has been used effectively to retrieve razor blades (Figure 1-34A). As prison doctors are well aware, razor blades can often be left to pass spontaneously, but many endoscopists feel uncomfortable doing this. Also, if the razor blade is wedged in the esophagus, efforts must be made to remove it. When the scope is advanced into the esophagus, the cup is dragged back over the shaft of the scope (Figure 1-34B). The endoscope with its rubber cup at the tip is positioned close to the razor blade, which is grasped with forceps or a snare (Figure 1-34C). The razor blade is then pulled against the tip of the scope, and the endoscope is withdrawn. The act of pulling the endoscope back causes the cup to form over the razor blade (Figure 1-34D), thereby protecting the wall of the esophagus and hypopharynx from the sharp edges.

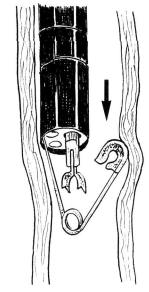

Figure 1-32. If the safety pin cannot be closed using the technique described in Figure 1-31, consider pulling the open pin against the tip of the scope, where the sharp point of the pin can be trapped and safely withdrawn.

Helicobacter pylori and Peptic Ulcers

The discovery that peptic ulcers are largely caused by bacterial infection is rapidly changing our management of this common condition. A majority of patients with duodenal ulcer and about half of patients with gastric ulcer have *Helicobacter pylori* infection. Because endoscopy and the processing of endoscopic biopsies is expensive compared with empiric antibiotic therapy, it has been suggested that all ulcer patients might be treated for *H. pylori* infection regardless of their *H. pylori* status. Graham and Rabeneck have recently suggested an algorithm for managing dyspepsia based on the presence or absence of *alarm features*, such as those that might indicate the presence of gastric cancer or a complication of peptic ulcer (Table 1-6). For those with alarm features, *H. pylori* serology or the urea breath test, or both, are performed. *H. pylori*–infected patients are treated with antibiotics; those without infection receive standard antisecretory therapy. If the symptoms remain unchanged after 2 weeks, endoscopy is performed.

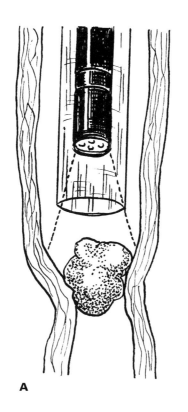

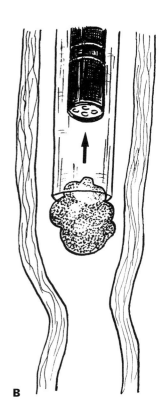

Figure 1-33. Meat bolus is (A) sucked into an overtube, (B) with which it is withdrawn.

A

B

Figure 1-34. Razor blade retrieval. A. A flexible rubber cup slips over the end of an endoscope. B. The cup is rolled back over the shaft of the endoscope. C. The endoscope, with the rubber cup retracted, is advanced into the esophagus, and the razor blade is grasped with a forceps or snare. D. The act of withdrawing the endoscope causes the cup to extend over and envelop the razor blade, which protects the wall of the esophagus.

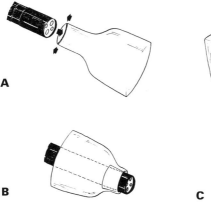

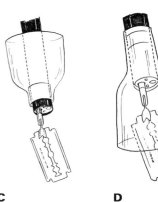

A

B

C

D

Table 1-6. Suggested algorithm for management of dyspepsia based on the presence or absence of "alarm features" and *Helicobacter pylori*

Prompt endoscopy	Endoscopy optional
Advanced age	Young patient
Long history	Short history
Weight loss	No weight loss
Anorexia	Normal appetite
GI bleeding/anemia	Normal hemoglobin
Persistent vomiting	No vomiting
Upper GI suggests cancer	Upper GI shows duodenal ulcer
	Nonsteroidal anti-inflammatory drug use

GI = gastrointestinal.
Source: Modified from DY Graham, L Rabeneck. Patients, payers and paradigm shifts: what to do about *Helicobacter pylori*. Am J Gastroenterol 1996;91:188.

Slide tests to detect *H. pylori* in gastric biopsies taken during endoscopy rely on the urease activity of the organism. A color change indicates the presence of *Helicobacter*. However, endoscopy is expensive. It is likely that in future the majority of patients will be screened for *Helicobacter* using serology (to detect antibodies) or carbon isotope– (C-13 or C-14) based breath tests. There is considerable interest in the association between *Helicobacter* and gastric cancer, as well as its role in causing unusual lymphomas (mucosa-associated lymphoid tissue—MALT) that regress with antibiotic therapy. Immunization against *Helicobacter* may one day become routine and relegate duodenal ulcers to the history books.

Suggested Reading

Esophageal Strictures

McClave SA, Brady PG, Wright RA, et al. Does fluoroscopic guidance for Maloney esophageal dilation impact on the clinical endpoint of therapy: relief of dysphagia and achievement of luminal patency. Gastrointest Endosc 1996;43:93.

Tulman AB, Boyce HW Jr. Complications of esophageal dilation and guidelines for their prevention. Gastrointest Endosc 1981;27:229.

Wesdorp ICE, Bartelman JFWM, den Hartog Jager FCA, et al. Results of conservative treatment of benign esophageal strictures: a follow-up study of 100 patients. Gastroenterology 1982;82:487.

Rigid Versus Balloon Dilators

Saeed ZA, Winchester CB, Ferro PS, et al. Prospective randomized comparison of polyvinyl bougies and through-the-scope balloons for dilation of peptic strictures of the esophagus. Gastrointest Endosc 1995;41:189.

Achalasia

Kadakia SC, Wong RKH. Graded pneumatic dilation using Rigiflex achalasia dilators in patients with primary esophageal achalasia. Am J Gastroenterol 1993;88:34.

Parkman HP, Reynolds JC, Ouyang A, et al. Pneumatic dilator or esophagomyotomy treatment for achalasia: clinical outcomes and cost analysis. Dig Dis Sci 1993;38:75.

Botulinum Toxin

Pasricha PJ, Ravich WJ, Hendrix TR, et al. Intrasphincteric botulinum toxin for the treatment of achalasia. N Engl J Med 1995;322:774.

Barrett's Esophagus

Avaska J, Miettinen M, Kivilaakso E. Adenocarcinoma arising in Barrett's esophagus. Dig Dis Sci 1989;34:1336.

Castell DO, Katzka DA. Barrett's esophagus: a continuing dilemma. Practical Gastroenterology 1995;19:22B.

Ortiz A, Martinez de Haro LF, Parrillo P, et al. Conservative treatment vs. antireflux surgery in Barrett's oesophagus: longterm results of a prospective study. Br J Surg 1996;83:274.

Provenzale D, Kemp AJ, Arora S, Wong JB. A guide for surveillance of patients with Barrett's esophagus. Am J Gastroenterol 1994;89:670.

Spechler SJ, Goyal RK. Barrett's esophagus. N Engl J Med 1986;315:362.

Weinstein WM, Ippoliti AF. The diagnosis of Barrett's esophagus: goblets, goblets, goblets [editorial]. Gastrointest Endosc 1996;44:91.

Metal Mesh Stents

Axelrad AM, Fleischer DE, Gomes M. Nitinol coil esophageal prothesis: advantages of removable self-expanding metal stents. Gastrointest Endosc 1996;43:161.

Bethge N, Sommer A, von Kleist D, Vakil N. A prospective trial of self-expanding metal stents in the palliation of malignant esophageal obstruction after failure of primary curative therapy. Gastrointest Endosc 1996;44:283.

Fleischer DE. Stents, cloggology and esophageal cancer [editorial]. Gastrointest Endosc 1996;43:258.

Kozarek RA, Ball TJ, Brandabur JJ, et al. Expandable versus conventional esophageal prostheses: easier insertion may not preclude subsequent stent-related problems. Gastrointest Endosc 1996;43:204.

Macken E, Gevers A, Hiele M, Rutgeerts P. Treatment of esophago-respiratory fistulas with a polyurethane-covered self-expanding metallic mesh stent. Gastrointest Endosc 1996;44:324.

Raijman I, Lalor E, Marcon NE. Photodynamic therapy for tumor ingrowth through an expandable esophageal stent. Gastrointest Endosc 1995;41:73.

Vermeijden JR, Bartelsman JFWM, Foekens P. Self-expanding metal stents for palliation of esophagocardial malignancies. Gastrointest Endosc 1995;41:58.

Wu WC, Katon RM, Saxon RR, et al. Silicon-covered self-expanding metallic stents for the palliation of malignant esophageal obstruction and esophago-respiratory fistulas: experience in 32 patients and a review of the literature. Gastrointest Endosc 1994;40:22.

Ablation of Obstructing Esophageal Tumors

Barr H, Krasner N. Prospective quality of life analysis after palliative photoablation for the treatment of malignant dysphagia. Cancer 1991;68:1660.

Bown SG. Palliation of malignant dysphagia: surgery, radiotherapy, laser, intubation alone or in combination? Gut 1991;32:841.

Hagenmuller F, Sander C, Sander R, et al. Laser and after-loading radiation with Ir[192]. In J Reimann, C Ell (eds), Lasers in Gastroenterology. Stuttgart, Germany: Georg Thieme Verlag, 1989;105.

Jensen DM, Machichado G, Randall G, et al. Comparison of low power YAG laser and Bicap tumor probe for palliation of esophageal cancer strictures. Gastroenterology 1988;94:1263.

Lightdale CJ, Heier SK, Marcon NE, et al. Photodynamic therapy with porfimer sodium versus thermal ablation therapy with Nd:YAG laser for palliation of esophageal cancer: a multicenter randomized trial. Gastrointest Endosc 1995;42:507.

Loizou LA, Grigg D, Atkinson M, et al. A prospective comparison of laser therapy and intubation in endoscopic palliation for malignant dysphagia. Gastroenterology 1991;100:1303.

Payne-James J, Spiller RC, Misiewicz JJ, Silk DB. Use of ethanol-induced tumour necrosis to palliate dysphagia in patients with oesophago-gastric cancer. Gastrointest Endosc 1990;36:43.

Renwick P, Whitton V, Moghissi K. Combined endoscopic laser therapy and brachytherapy for palliation of oesophageal carcinoma. Gut 1992;33:435.

How Should Endoscopic Methods of Hemostasis Be Used?

Chung SCS, Leung JWC, Steele RJC, et al. Endoscopic injection of adrenalin for actively bleeding ulcers: a randomized trial. BMJ 1988;296:1631.

Laine L. Multipolar electrocoagulation in the treatment of peptic ulcers with non-bleeding visible vessels. Ann Intern Med 1989;110:510.

Laine L, Stein C, Sharma V. A prospective outcome study of patients with clot in an ulcer and the effect of irrigation. Gastrointest Endosc 1996;43:107.

Llach J, Bordas JM, Salmeron JM, et al. A prospective randomized trial of heater probe thermocoagulation versus injection therapy in peptic ulcer hemorrhage. Gastrointest Endosc 1996;43:117.

Matthewson K, Swain CP, Bland M, et al. Randomized comparison of Nd-YAG laser, heater probe and no endoscopic therapy for bleeding peptic ulcer. Gastroenteroscopy 1990;98:1239.

NIH Consensus Development Conference. Therapeutic endoscopy and bleeding ulcers. JAMA 1989;262:1369.

Swain CP, Bown SG, Stoney DW, et al. Controlled trial of argon laser photocoagulation in bleeding peptic ulcers. Lancet 1981;8259:1313.

Swain CP, Kirkham JS, Salmon PR, et al. Controlled trial of Nd-YAG laser photocoagulation in bleeding peptic ulcers. Lancet 1986;8490:1113.

Esophageal and Gastric Varices

Korula J. Endoscopic therapy of bleeding varices: do studies in animal models give us the answers we need? Gastrointest Endosc 1995;41:265.

Laine L, Cook D. Endoscopic ligation compared with sclerotherapy for treatment of esophageal variceal bleeding. A meta-analysis. Ann Intern Med 1995;123:280.

Stiegmann GV, Goff JS, Sun JH, et al. Endoscopic variceal ligation: an alternative to sclerotherapy. Gastrointest Endosc 1989;35:431.

Urita Y, Kondo E, Muto M, et al. Combined endoscopic clipping and injection sclerotherapy for esophageal varices. Gastrointest Endosc 1995;43:140.

Percutaneous Gastrostomy and Percutaneous Jejunostomy

Ching AX. Complications of the skin level gastrostomy device. Gastrointest Endosc 1993;39:467.

Gauderer MWL. Long term gastric access: caveat medicus [editorial]. Gastrointest Endosc 1996;44:356.

Kozarek RA, Payne M, Barkin J, et al. Prospective multicenter evaluation of an initially replaced button gastrostomy. Gastrointest Endosc 1995;41:105.

Parasher VK, Abramowicz CJ, Bell C, et al. Successful placement of percutaneous gastrojejunostomy using a steerable guidewire—a modified, controlled "push" technique. Gastrointest Endosc 1995;44:52.

Railey DJ, Calleja GA, Barkin JS. Percutaneous endoscopic jejunostomy. Gastrointest Endosc Clin North Am 1992;2:223.

Wolfsen HC, Kozarek RA. Percutaneous endoscopic gastrostomy: ethical considerations. Gastrointest Endosc Clin North Am 1992;2:259.

Ingested Foreign Bodies

Ginsberg GG. Management of ingested foreign objects and food bolus impactions. Gastrointest Endosc 1995;41:33.

Webb WA. Management of foreign bodies of the upper GI tract: update. Gastrointest Endosc 1995;41:39.

Helicobacter pylori *and Peptic Ulcers*

Graham DY, Rabeneck L. Patients, payers and paradigm shifts: what to do about *Helicobacter pylori*. Am J Gastroenterol 1996;91:188.

Peura DA. *Helicobacter pylori*: a diagnostic dilemma and a dilemma of diagnosis [editorial]. Gastroenterology 1995;109:313.

Peura DA. *Helicobacter pylori* and ulcerogenesis (a review). Am J Med 1996;100:19S.

Tytgat GNJ, Lee A, Graham DY, et al. The role of infectious agents in peptic ulcer disease. Gastroenterol Int 1993;6:76.

2

Colon Problems and Solutions

Is Colonoscopy More Difficult in Women?

It often seems to experienced endoscopists that colonoscopy is technically more difficult in women patients than in men, as judged by the success rates for cecal intubation. Is this true, and, if so, what is the reason for the difference? Saunders and colleagues from Christopher Williams' Endoscopy Unit at St. Mark's Hospital in London have recently studied these questions. In a retrospective review of a single expert operator's experience of 2,194 colonoscopies between 1988 and 1993, 31% of examinations in women were considered technically difficult compared with 16% in men. The most common difficulty encountered was looping of the colonoscope due to a long or excessively mobile colon. To investigate the differences between women and men more scientifically, barium enema examinations (183 women, 162 men) were studied to determine colon length and mobility using blinded observers (Figure 2-1). Total colon length was greater in women (median, 155 cm, compared with 145 cm for men) despite their generally smaller stature. The principal difference was in the length of the transverse colon: The median length in the women was 48 cm, compared with 40 cm in the men. The transverse colon reached the true pelvis in more women (62%) than men (26%). The authors of this study concluded that the impression that colonoscopy is technically more challenging in women may be due to their inherently longer colons.

Polyps

The technique of colonoscopic polypectomy is well established. Difficulties arise, however, when large polyps are encountered. These troublesome polyps can be divided into two main groups: pedunculated and broad-based. Pedunculated polyps have the classic mushroom appearance (Figure 2-2); they are usually tubular or tubulovillous adenomas. The larger the size of the head of the polyp (> 2 cm), the greater is the chance that it will contain a focus of malignancy (adenocarcinoma). If this malignancy is confined to the head (i.e., without gross venous or lymphatic invasion),

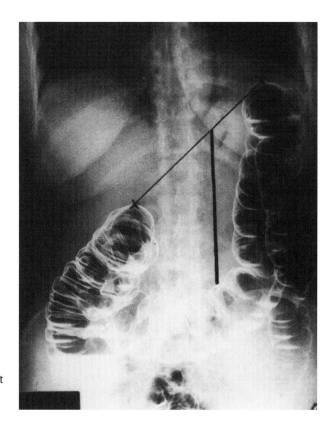

Figure 2-1. Double-contrast barium enema showing measurement of transverse colon mobility. (Reprinted with permission from BP Saunders, M Fukumoto, S Halligan, et al. Why is colonoscopy more difficult in women? Gastrointest Endosc 1996;43:124.)

polypectomy is curative. Broad-based polyps that may take up a significant part of the circumference of the bowel wall are usually villous adenomas. Because these, too, have malignant potential, they demand careful and definitive management.

Large Pedunculated Polyps

Large polyps with a stalk present a technical problem to snare. It may prove impossible (or seem impossibly difficult) to negotiate the loop of the snare over the head of the polyp. Obviously, a minisnare is unlikely to do the job. If the usual tricks fail, such as bending the loop of the snare back on itself (over the polyp head), consideration should be given to removing the polyp head piecemeal (Figure 2-3). Chunks of the polyp can be removed until the head reaches a manageable size. It is important to ensure that a generous amount of stalk is sent to the pathologist for study because the determination of whether or not carcinoma in situ has spread locally has important therapeutic implications. Once a snare is negotiated

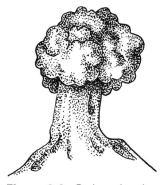

Figure 2-2. Pedunculated polyp.

over the polyp head, the polyp can be quite difficult to remove, so it is best not to attempt this unless you intend to go ahead with the polypectomy. Thick stalks often contain large blood vessels and therefore carry increased risk of hemorrhage from the procedure. Given that it is harder to achieve a high current density during snare polypectomy when the stalk is thick (rather than thin), great care has to be taken to ensure that adequate cautery has been achieved before the stalk is transected. Some endoscopists prefer to use higher-than-normal current settings for their electrocautery. Others prefer to use more "cut" in blended form than usual, to prevent the snare from adhering to the stalk. Whatever combination is used, a rapid cut should be avoided. If excessive coagulation occurs, and the snare becomes embedded in the stalk, there is little alternative but to close the snare and transect it. Further electrocautery is unlikely to help. The tissue surrounding the snare has already been desiccated (dried out) and cannot be transected further by heating.

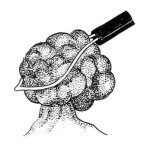

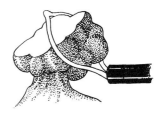

Several techniques have been advocated to reduce the bleeding risk from large pedunculated polyps (see Figure 2-2) during polypectomy. The first is to inject the stalk with 1:10,000 solution of epinephrine (adrenaline) solution using a sclerotherapy needle (Figure 2-4A). Whatever volume it takes to cause the stalk to swell and blanch (it often assumes a purplish discoloration) should be injected, usually 2–5 ml (Figure 2-4B). Some authors suggest mixing the epinephrine with hypertonic (1.8%) saline. This hypertonic medium causes osmotic swelling of the tissue of the stalk, which (at least theoretically) should increase interstitial pressure and may reduce postpolypectomy hemorrhage. Injected epinephrine does not appear to have adverse systemic effects. Another safety maneuver is to use a double-channel colonoscope and pass two snares to surround the stalk (Figure 2-5). The lower snare is left loose while the upper one is used to perform the electrocautery. Should hemorrhage occur when the stalk is transected, the lower snare is immediately tightened to compress the bleeding vessel. The remaining stalk can then be cauterized to effect hemostasis. Although an attractive concept, this technique is more cumbersome than injecting the polyp base. For one thing, a double-channel colonoscope is required; these are not universally available, even in some large endoscopy units. Also, it can be maddeningly difficult to obtain suitable orientation of both snares. If, despite these precautions, immediate hemorrhage occurs from a polypectomy site, several remedies exist. When the end of the stalk remains visible (which is likely to be the bleeding site), it can be grasped using the snare and cautery applied. If, as is usually the case, only a crater is left, and a spurting artery is visible at its base, local cautery can be applied using the partially retracted snare tip. If time allows, a heater probe or similar cautery device can be passed and appropriate therapy applied. Alternatively, local injection of the offending vessel with epinephrine can be equally effective.

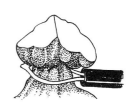

Figure 2-3. Piecemeal snare resection of a polyp head.

The job is not finished until the resected polyp has been recovered for histologic analysis. A large polyp cannot be aspirated through the suction channel into a suction trap. If you try to remove it solely by suction against

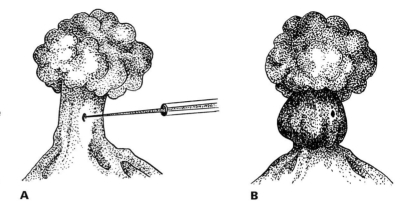

Figure 2-4. A. Injecting the stalk of a large polyp with epinephrine solution.
B. When 2–5 ml of epinephrine have been injected, the stalk swells and is often discolored.

the tip of the colonoscope, it is almost always dislodged before it exits the rectum. If the loop of the snare can be fitted comfortably around the polyp head and tightened just enough to ensure a firm grip, this usually does the trick. To reduce the risk of accidental dislodgement, the snare should be pulled back so that the polyp head is held snugly against the scope tip during withdrawal. If the colon needs to remain visible for inspection, the basket catheter or snare can be allowed to trail the endoscope tip by a few centimeters. Three-pronged graspers are useful if the polyp head is not excessively large. Another ingenious solution to the problem has been the polyp retrieval basket, a little net on a snare that can be used to "fish" for the resected tissue.

If the resected polyp is lost, colonic lavage, either through the scope using a syringe of saline or by enema immediately following scope removal, can coax the missing polyp from hiding. If, as often happens, the polyp is dislodged during attempted removal through the anal canal, it can often be retrieved by digital rectal examination.

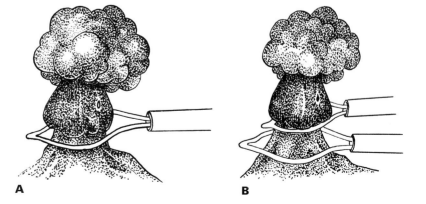

Figure 2-5. Using a double-channel colonoscope, (A) one and then (B) two snares are advanced around the stalk of a large polyp.

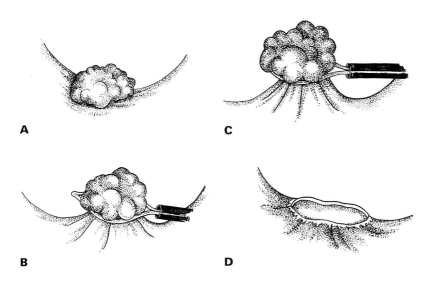

A

B

C

D

Figure 2-6. A. A sessile polyp. B. A snare is placed around the base of the polyp. C. The polyp is lifted away from the bowel wall ("tented") by the tightened snare. Tenting the tissue to pull it away from the bowel wall reduces the likelihood of an electrocautery burn. D. Using electrocautery, the polyp is burned off, leaving a shallow crater.

Broad-Based (Sessile) Polyps

Large sessile polyps are often villous adenomas. Some come to light because of their tendency to cause watery diarrhea rich in potassium (causing hypokalemia). Sessile polyps are more difficult to remove in their entirety than pedunculated ones, because they have a broad base extending right down to the bowel wall. Great caution is needed when applying electrocautery near the bowel wall, to avoid a transmural burn or perforation. Often the tissue has to be removed piecemeal. Tenting the tissue to pull it away from the bowel wall reduces the likelihood of a burn (Figure 2-6). Injection with epinephrine in this situation is rarely helpful because the soft polyp is not firm enough to retain the fluid and increase tissue tension. Submucosal injection of saline to raise up the polyp may increase the safety of subsequent snare excision (Figure 2-7).

Carpet polyps, which occupy a significant area of the colon wall, represent another treatment problem. Thermal ablation by heater probe using a sweeping motion, back and forth across the surface of the "carpet," may be a suitable alternative to surgical resection (Figure 2-8). Sometimes, sessile polyps are floppy and tend to drape over folds (*saddle* polyps) (Figure 2-9). Usually, these can be tented and snared without difficulty.

Large villous polyps are difficult to remove in their entirety. Their potential for malignancy makes laser or other thermal ablation of residual tissue problematic in younger patients, who may need segmental resection or sleeve surgical resection to ensure that a potentially malignant lesion is completely removed. In elderly or debilitated patients who represent poor

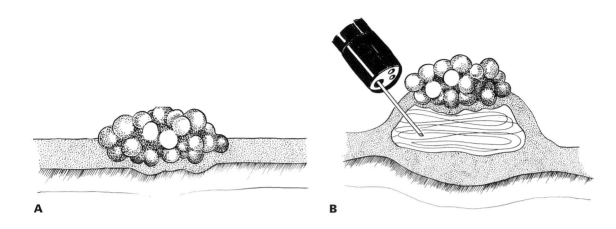

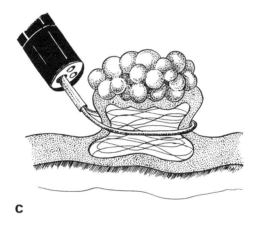

Figure 2-7. The sequence of results of injecting saline submucosally to raise up a polyp for subsequent snare excision. A. A large sessile polyp. B. Saline is injected into the submucosa to lift the polyp clear of the sero-muscular wall of the colon. C. After the "saline lift," the elevated base is snared and snare cautery is performed in the standard way.

risks for such surgery, palliative thermal ablation may keep a patient asymptomatic for long periods, especially when bleeding or obstruction has been a problem.

Small Polyps

As Waye has pointed out, there are six approaches to small polyps, defined as being 5 mm or less in diameter.

1. *Leave it alone.* The majority of small polyps in the rectum (80%) are hyperplastic, whereas 70% of those in the right colon are adenomas. Hyperplastic polyps in the rectum are rarely associated with adenomas more proximally, but because these two types of polyp are impossible to distinguish by eye, biopsy for histology is necessary. Adenomas in the left

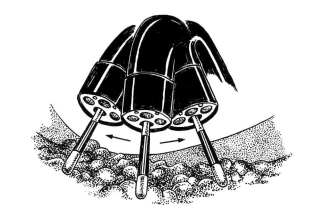

Figure 2-8. Using a sweeping motion with a thermal probe is one way to deal with a carpet polyp.

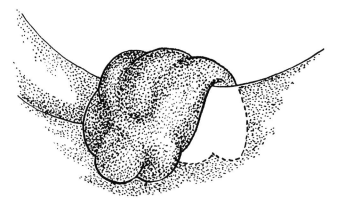

Figure 2-9. A saddle polyp, so called because it straddles a fold like a horse's saddle.

colon are markers for adenomas in the rest of the colon. Hyperplastic polyps in the rectum may flatten and disappear with air insufflation.

2. *Hot biopsy forceps.* Employ insulated cups to grasp tissue, with only the portion grasped by the jaws being exposed to cutting current (Figure 2-10). The polyp tissue is therefore undamaged and can be sent for histologic analysis. A zone of whitening (tissue desiccation) is seen at the polyp base. Hot biopsy technique has received adverse publicity because of delayed hemorrhage, which results from sloughing of necrotic tissue. Perforation is also a potential risk of hot biopsy technique, although reports have been rare. A concern about hot biopsy is that all the neoplastic tissue may not be removed, especially if a large polyp (i.e., > 5 mm) is the target. This is a good reason to ensure that only polyps of a diameter larger than 5 mm are treated using this technique.

3. *Snare-cautery technique.* This is the well-established technique of grasping a polyp with a snare and applying current. Submucosal injection

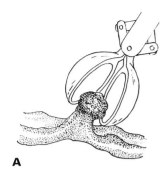

A

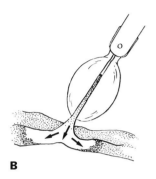

B

Figure 2-10. Hot biopsy forceps being used to remove a small colonic polyp. A. A small polyp is captured within the cups of specially modified forceps. B. With the forceps closed, current is applied to transect the polyp base. To reduce the risk of thermal injury from leaking current (arrows), the polyp is pulled away from the bowel wall as cautery is applied.

of saline to elevate the polyp may render this technique safer. Because the incidence of complications of snare cautery is low anyway, this is probably overkill.

4. *Multiple bites with forceps (cold biopsy).* This is an unreliable method for removing polyps because it is difficult to ensure that all the adenomatous tissue has been removed. One published study estimated that polypoid tissue remained at the biopsy site in 29% of cases.

5. *Local cautery.* The tip of a snare can be used to coagulate multiple small polyps at a single sitting, but tissue is not retrieved. This is probably an acceptable technique if the histology of the polyps is already known.

6. *Snare excision without cautery.* Although endoscopists have always been nervous about the possible sequelae of transecting polyps without adequate cautery, the incidence of postpolypectomy bleeding is quite small. The recommended technique is to pull back on the polyp, creating a neck, which is guillotined. Waye recommends this technique, which he has used with only rare instances of bleeding that were easily treated with local electrocautery (Waye prefers the term *garotte* to *guillotine*).

Surveillance Colonoscopy After Polypectomy

The objective of postpolypectomy surveillance is to reduce the risk of developing colorectal cancer. When considering surveillance in patients with prior polyps, we must appreciate the following:

1. Certain postpolypectomy patients are at increased risk of colon cancer and therefore require surveillance.
2. The risk of colon cancer is not the same for all patients.
3. The interval between the formation of a polyp and its transformation into a cancer is considerable (years).

In developing strategies for colon cancer surveillance, we also need to address such questions as what factors may predict recurrence of polyps, how frequently surveillance should be performed, the risks and costs of repeated colonoscopy, patient compliance, and so forth. Outcome analysis will be extremely important in determining the future pattern of postpolypectomy surveillance.

In these days of health care cutbacks, cost-benefit issues cannot be ignored. Colonoscopy has been shown repeatedly to be the investigation of choice. It is more sensitive than contrast studies for detecting small colon polyps, and it affords the opportunity to biopsy and remove most polyps at the time of the examination. What data support the use of colonoscopy as a means of colon cancer reduction? The National Polyp Study addressed the hypothesis that removing all polyps from the colon in a well-defined population would reduce the incidence of colorectal cancer.

In this study, 1,418 patients had total colonoscopy during which one or more adenomatous polyps were removed. These patients underwent periodic surveillance colonoscopy for a mean of 5.9 years. Five early (asymptomatic) cancers were detected by colonoscopy during the follow-up period, which was only 10–24% of the expected incidence based on comparison with reference groups. Only one-fourth of the highest expected incidence of colon cancer was seen in patients whose adenomatous polyps were removed during the study.

How often should colonoscopic surveillance be performed? The 1,418 patients in the National Polyp Study were randomized to receive follow-up colonoscopy at 1 and 3 years, or at 3 years only. Forty-two percent of patients in the 1- and 3-year follow-up group developed adenomas, compared with 32% in the group examined only at 3 years. The number of patients who developed *advanced adenomas* (> 1 cm diameter, high-grade dysplasia, or invasive carcinoma) was identical in both groups (3.3%). It was concluded that colonoscopy performed at 3 years after polyp resection detects new lesions as effectively as more aggressive surveillance (at 1 and 3 years). Additional information available from the National Polyp Study included the observations that recurrence of adenomas was more likely if the initial polyps contained villous tissue, were multiple, or if the patients were men, older than 50 years, or had a family history of colorectal cancer. This study also suggests that it takes on average 10 years for an adenomatous polyp to progress to cancer. J.H. Bond of the American College of Gastroenterology has developed a practice guideline, "Diagnosis, Treatment and Surveillance for Patients with Non-familial Colorectal Polyps," which has been endorsed by the American Gastroenterological Association and the American Society for Gastrointestinal Endoscopy. Its recommendations include the following:

1. Complete colonoscopy should be performed at the time of polypectomy to detect and resect all synchronous adenomas. Additional clearing examinations may be required after resections of large sessile adenomas or multiple adenomas to ensure complete resection.
2. Repeat colonoscopy to check for missed synchronous and metachronous adenomas is performed within 3 years for most patients with a single or only a few adenomas, provided that they have had a high-quality initial examination.
3. Selected patients with multiple adenomas, or those who have had a suboptimal initial examination, might require colonoscopy at 1 and 4 years.
4. After one negative 3-year follow-up examination result, subsequent surveillance intervals may be increased to 5 years.
5. The presence of severe or high-grade dysplasia in a resected polyp does not, per se, modify recommendations 1 through 4.
6. If complete colonoscopy is not possible, flexible sigmoidoscopy plus double-contrast barium enema is an acceptable alternative.
7. Because patients undergoing resection of a single small tubular ade-

noma (< 1 cm) do not have increased risk of subsequent cancer, follow-up surveillance is *not* indicated.

8. Surveillance should be individualized according to age and comorbidity of the patient, and it should be discontinued when it appears unlikely that continued follow-up is capable of prolonging life expectancy.

What data are available on the cost-benefit issue? Ransohoff argues that resection of small adenomas is unlikely to cause a significant reduction in colon cancer mortality. Because perhaps as many as 50% of adults over the age of 50 have small adenomas, and few of those will develop cancers, the cost of screening this population may be prohibitive. It might cost as much as $300,000 per life saved to operate a surveillance program for patients aged 50 years and over, assuming an examination every 3 years for 30 years. The costs of surveillance increase markedly when patients with false-positive fecal occult blood test results are included. Given the significant morbidity and mortality from colorectal cancer (about 150,000 new cases per year in the United States), postpolypectomy surveillance is an issue that cannot be ignored. At present, some patients have excessive surveillance, whereas others, who may benefit more, are lost to follow-up. Uniform guidelines are needed to ensure that every patient has the best possible chance to avoid developing colon cancer.

Tattooing for Identification

One way to identify the site of prior polypectomy for later follow-up is by submucosal injection of India ink (up to 0.5 ml of autoclaved 1:10 saline dilution) with a sclerotherapy-type injection needle. Williams has suggested that, for the best results, less than 1 ml of ink should be used and the needle should be advanced just under the surface and parallel to it. India ink injection has been used for many years to mark lesions for subsequent inspection at surgery. Although generally regarded as safe, India ink injection carries the potential for introducing infection and provoking an inflammatory response. Colonic abscess, fat necrosis, phlegmonous gastritis, and focal peritonitis have been attributed to this technique. Because the ink may become contaminated after autoclaving (i.e., before use in the clinical setting), it is recommended that a 0.22-µm filter be positioned between the syringe and the sclerotherapy needle to provide a bacteriostatic filter that excludes all living bacteria and fungi.

Colonic Pseudo-Obstruction (Ogilvie's Syndrome)

Colonic pseudo-obstruction (CPO) is a nonobstructive dilatation of the colon that is associated with a large number of medical conditions and the

Table 2-1. Common associations with colonic pseudo-obstruction

Drugs
   Narcotics
   Phenothiazines
   Anticholinergics
   Benzodiazepines
   Calcium channel blockers
   Cytotoxic agents
Metabolic
   Hypokalemia
   Hyponatremia
   Hypernatremia
   Hypocalcemia
   Hypercalcemia
   Hypomagnesemia
   Hypothyroidism
   Diabetes mellitus
   Porphyria
Sepsis
Surgery
Trauma
   Hip fracture in the elderly
   Multiple injuries
Anesthesia
Neurologic
   Subarachnoid hemorrhage
   Epidural anesthesia
   Parkinsonism
   Spinal cord disease
Mechanical ventilation
Renal
   Renal failure or dialysis
Neoplasm
   Invasion of lumbar sympathetic nerves
   Paraneoplastic syndromes
   Carcinomatosis

use of certain groups of drugs (Table 2-1). Although often asymptomatic, CPO may lead to colonic (usually cecal) perforation in a small number of patients. The endoscopist is usually called in to provide colonic decompression. Surprisingly little is known about the pathophysiology of CPO, but the typical patient is elderly with multiorgan failure and sepsis or in postoperative intensive care receiving narcotics, anticholinergics, phenothiazines, and other drugs. Although onset can be rapid, the usual course is slow progression over 3–7 days. The abdomen becomes distended and tympanitic. Pain is rare, and palpation usually fails to locate tenderness. Plain abdominal radiographic films show modest to massive distention of the colon; the abnormality is often limited to the cecum and right colon. The absence of air-fluid levels militates against the presence of mechanical obstruction. Bowel sounds are usually preserved. The diagnosis of CPO is rarely in doubt, but if there is any suspicion that an acute or subacute mechanical obstruction may be present, a contrast study should be performed. The advice of the radiologist should be obtained regarding choice of contrast medium (barium versus water-soluble).

The goal of treatment in CPO is to reduce the diameter of the colon and thereby reduce the risk of perforation, which is said to increase when the cecum is more than 12 cm (some say > 10 cm) in diameter. The rate of dilatation is also important. A rapidly dilating colon should be cause for great concern and urgent intervention. When a colon dilates slowly to 12 cm or greater in diameter and remains dilated for longer than 24 hours, prophylactic endoscopic decompression should be considered. A number of conservative measures, however, can be taken to improve the chances of spontaneous colon decompression:

1. If not already fasting, the patient should be given nothing by mouth and a nasogastric tube placed for suction.
2. Electrolyte, acid-base, and fluid imbalances should be corrected.
3. Drugs that may have precipitated the problem, especially narcotics and phenothiazines, should be discontinued whenever possible.
4. Underlying sepsis should be treated.
5. The patient should be repositioned regularly. The simple act of turning the patient supine may be enough to induce passage of flatus.
6. A rectal (flatus) tube should be placed (on low wall suction).
7. Tap water enemas may be helpful (but cathartics should not be administered).

Some authors recommend the routine use of broad-spectrum parenteral antibiotics as prophylaxis in case the colon perforates. Conservative therapy requires regular review to look for signs of peritoneal irritation, increasing distention, pain, fever, and other signs that perforation is imminent or has already occurred. Conservative measures provide adequate therapy in the majority of cases of CPO. The use of drugs known to improve colonic motility (prokinetic agents) has been largely anecdotal, although guanethidine (a sympathetic blocking agent) has recently shown promise in a small case series.

Colonoscopic Decompression in Colonic Pseudo-Obstruction

This technique was first described in 1977 and has seen increasing use ever since. The indications for colonoscopic decompression are persistent abdominal distention, especially if painful; failure to respond to conservative measures after 24–48 hours; and (possibly) cecal diameter greater than 12 cm. Rex feels that there is a "12-cm myth," which belies the fact that, in some cases, the colon may not perforate until it reaches 25 cm. As he states, however, if the "magic" diameter of 12 cm brings the patient to the attention of a gastroenterologist, it is a myth worth preserving. **Colonoscopy is absolutely contraindicated when there is evidence of impending or actual perforation.**

The colonoscopic examination for decompression is usually performed without formal bowel preparation because the contents of the colon are often liquid. Insertion of the colonoscope with minimal insufflation is appropriate. When the distended section of colon is entered, some air should be aspirated because this deflates the bowel and allows further passage of the instrument. Sometimes the act of passing the colonoscope allows the patient to expel gas, but because this is usually accompanied by liquid stool, the endoscopist should choose a strategically safe place to stand (out of the line of fire).

Rex collated data from 24 published studies and found that 69% of patients (201 of 292) were judged to have been successfully decompressed by initial colonoscopy. However, 40% of patients who appeared to have been decompressed successfully suffered at least one recurrence requiring repeat colonoscopy. For this reason, most endoscopists prefer to place a decompression tube at the time of colonoscopy for CPO. There are several ways to do this. One is to drag a tube around the colon. A suture tied to the end of the decompression tube is grasped with biopsy forceps exiting the colonoscope. The tube is then dragged along as the colonoscope advances, finally being released in the cecum. In addition to being rather cumbersome, this technique has a distinct disadvantage in that the tube may be dragged back (by friction) as the colonoscope is withdrawn. The currently favored technique is to advance the tube over an endoscopically placed guidewire that has been left in the right colon as the colonoscope is withdrawn (Figure 2-11).

A variety of decompression tubes are available (all 480 cm long) with sizes (circumferences) ranging from 7 to 14 Fr (Figure 2-12). In the author's experience, decompression tubes less than 10 Fr clog quickly and are often ineffective. The tubes have side holes to aid suction. To ensure that the wire and tube are correctly placed, this procedure should be performed under fluoroscopy whenever practical. CPO is often treated in the intensive care setting, where mobile fluoroscopy (C-arm) is usually available.

Modifications of standard decompression tube placement include using a stiff guidewire (e.g., Savary guidewire) and a colon-straightening overtube. It is important to flush the decompression tube periodically (e.g., every 6 hours) with saline or sterile water to maintain patency. Usually, the tube can be withdrawn after a few days, although the patient is likely to expel it when colonic motility returns. Colonoscopy for decompression of CPO carries an increased risk of complications, including perforation. For this reason, considerable endoscopic skill and experience are desirable.

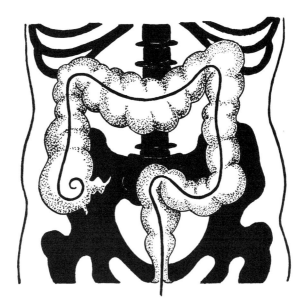

Figure 2-11. Decompression of a colonic pseudo-obstruction. A decompression tube is advanced over an endoscopically placed guidewire that has been left in the right colon as the colonoscope is withdrawn.

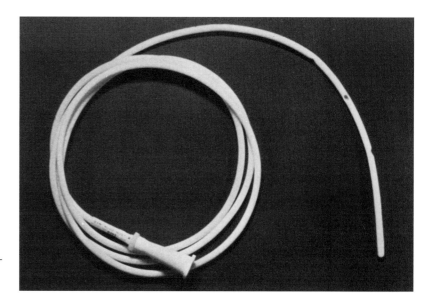

Figure 2-12. A decompression tube for treatment of colonic pseudo-obstruction.

If endoscopic decompression fails, and CPO persists or worsens, surgery may be necessary. Unless perforation has occurred, tube cecostomy is the usual procedure performed. Percutaneous and endoscopic cecostomy have both been described as alternative means of cecal decompression, but neither has gained widespread acceptance.

Table 2-2. Probability of finding carcinoma in colectomy specimens from ulcerative colitis patients

Dysplasia grade	Immediate colectomy	Colectomy after some follow-up
High	42% (10/24)	32% (15/47)
Low	19% (3/16)	8% (17/204)

Source: Modified from CN Bernstein, F Shanahan, WM Weinstein. Are we telling patients the truth about surveillance colonoscopy in ulcerative colitis? Lancet 1994;343:71.

Surveillance Colonoscopy in Ulcerative Colitis

Ulcerative colitis (UC) carries an increased risk of adenocarcinoma of the colon, estimated at 7% after 20 years and 7–14% at 25 years. The issue of colonoscopic surveillance in UC remains controversial, however. How often should surveillance be performed? What is the significance of dysplasia? Who needs colectomy? These questions have provoked considerable debate. Dysplasia is a histologic abnormality that is believed to suggest or predict progression to overt malignancy.

Bernstein et al. assessed the predictive value of high- and low-grade dysplasia in colonic biopsies in patients with ulcerative colitis who underwent colectomy (Table 2-2). Of 25 carcinomas discovered, 11 (44%) were at Dukes C stage, or worse. Two of the three patients with low-grade dysplasia who were found to have carcinomas had Dukes B lesions. Colectomy has been recommended for high-grade dysplasia and for dysplasia-associated lesions or masses. Of concern, 29% of 55 UC patients followed with low-grade dysplasia subsequently developed high-grade dysplasia, dysplasia-associated lesions or masses, or carcinoma. Patients undergoing colonoscopy for UC surveillance whose biopsies were negative for dysplasia had about a 2.5% chance of progression toward cancer. However, the risk in those with definite biopsies was 18–28%. When high-grade dysplasia was present, there was a 40% chance that cancer was present; half of those cancers were advanced.

How often should surveillance be performed? A family history of colon cancer or duration of UC greater than 20 years mandates a formal surveillance program. Some start surveillance as early as 8 years from initial diagnosis. The standard recommendation of two to four endoscopic biopsies for every 10 cm of colon is somewhat arbitrary as there is bound to be a sampling error. Multiple biopsies, however, should increase the overall yield of surveillance colonoscopy. Until genetic and other cell marker studies allow accurate stratification of risk, some experts advocate prophylactic colectomy for all patients with pancolitis in UC of greater than 20 years' duration.

Suggested Reading

Is Colonoscopy More Difficult in Women?

Saunders BP, Fukumoto M, Halligan S, et al. Why is colonoscopy more difficult in women? Gastrointest Endosc 1996;43:124.

Polyps

Binmoeller KF, Bohnacker S, Seifert F, et al. Endoscopic snare excision of "giant" colorectal polyps. Gastrointest Endosc 1996;43:183

Neugut AI, Bassam A-R. Lessons from the follow-up of large colorectal adenomomas: BE or not BE, that is the question [editorial]. Am J Gastroenterol 1996;91:420.

Tappero G, Gaia E, De Giuli P, et al. Cold snare-excision of small colorectal polyps. Gastroenterology 1992;38:310.

Waye JD. Endoscopic treatment of adenoma. World J Surg 1991;15:14.

Waye JD. How big is too big [editorial]? Gastrointest Endosc 1996;43:256.

Waye JD, Lewis BS, Yessayan S. Colonoscopy: a prospective report of complications. J Clin Gastroenterol 1992;15:347.

Waye JD, Lewis BS, Frankel A, Geller SA. Small colon polyps. Am J Gastroenterol 1988;83:120.

Surveillance Colonoscopy After Polypectomy

Bond JH. Polyp guidelines: diagnosis, treatment and surveillance for patients with non-familial colorectal polyps. Ann Intern Med 1993;119:836.

Lieberman DA. Colon cancer screening: what is the question [editorial]? Gastrointest Endosc 1996;44:203.

Winawer SJ, Zauber AG, Ho MN, et al. Prevention of colorectal cancer by colonoscopic polypectomy. N Engl J Med 1993;329:1977.

Winawer SJ, Zauber AG, O'Brien MJ, et al. Randomized comparison of surveillance intervals after colonoscopic removal of newly diagnosed adenomatous polyps. N Engl J Med 1993;328:901.

Tattooing for Identification

Coman E, Brandt LJ, Brenner S, et al. Fat necrosis and inflammatory pseudotumor due to endoscopic tattooing of the colon. Gastrointest Endosc 1991;37:65.

Park SI, Genta RS, Romeo DP, Weesner RE. Colonic abscess and focal peritonitis secondary to India ink tattooing of the colon. Gastrointest Endosc 1991;37:68.

Salomon P, Berner JS, Waye JD. Endoscopic India ink injection: a method for preparation, sterilization and administration. Gastrointest Endosc 1993;39:803.

Colonic Pseudo-Obstruction (Ogilvie's Syndrome) and Colonic Decompression

Duh Q-Y, Way LW. Diagnostic laparoscopy and laparoscopic cecostomy for colonic pseudo-obstruction. Dis Colon Rectum 1993;36:65.

Geller A, Petersen BT, Gostout CJ. Endoscopic decompression for acute colonic pseudo-obstruction. Gastrointest Endosc 1996;44:144.

Harig JM, Fumo DE, Loo FD, et al. Treatment of acute non-toxic megacolon during colonoscopy: tube placement versus simple decompression. Gastrointest Endosc 1988;34:23.

Ponsky JL. Colonoscopic Decompression. In JL Pinsky (ed), Atlas of Surgical Endoscopy. St. Louis: Mosby, 1992;231.

Vantrappen G. Acute colonic pseudo-obstruction. Lancet 1993;341:152.

Surveillance Colonoscopy in Ulcerative Colitis

Baillie J. Gastrointestinal Endoscopy: Basic Principles and Practice. Oxford, England: Butterworth-Heinemann, 1992.

Bernstein CN, Shanahan F, Weinstein WM. Are we telling patients the truth about surveillance colonoscopy in ulcerative colitis? Lancet 1994;343:71.

Blackstone MO, Riddell RH, Rogers BH, et al. Dysplasia-associated lesion or mass (DALM) detected by colonoscopy in longstanding ulcerative colitis: an indication for colectomy. Gastroenterology 1981;80:366.

Riddell RH, Goldman H, Ransohoff DF, et al. Dysplasia in inflammatory bowel disease: standardized classification with provisional clinical applications. Hum Pathol 1983;14:931.

Rubin CE, Haggitt RC, Burmer GC. DNA aneuploidy in colonic biopsies predicts future development of dysplasia in ulcerative colitis. Gastroenterology 1992;103:1611.

3

Endoscopic Retrograde Cholangiopancreatography Problems and Solutions

Periampullary Diverticula

Many endoscopists consider the presence of duodenal diverticula a major obstacle to successful endoscopic retrograde cholangiopancreatography (ERCP). This need not be the case. Despite the displacement of the normal papillary structure by periampullary diverticula, it is usually possible to identify and cannulate an orifice for ERCP.

It is now well established that diverticula in the vicinity of the duodenal papilla encourage the formation of bile duct stones. The mechanism for this is uncertain, but reasonable hypotheses include (1) disordered motility and (2) retrograde bacterial colonization of the biliary tree resulting from bacterial overgrowth within the diverticula. As with most diverticula in the GI tract, these structures are not true diverticula because they lack all the layers of the bowel wall. Accordingly, they are more accurately described as *pseudodiverticula*. The injudicious use of guidewires and cannulae within diverticula may result in retroperitoneal perforation.

When periampullary diverticula are encountered at ERCP, which is increasingly likely as the age of the patient increases, it is important to approach the problem in an organized fashion. First, the area should be minutely inspected for an obvious papilla. It is not unusual for the papillary structure to run along one wall of the diverticulum (Figure 3-1A), which may result in the orifice of the papilla being at an uncomfortable angle for cannulation. Dexterity with catheters and guidewires is essential for successful ERCP in this situation. A variety of maneuvers can be performed safely. Once deep cannulation has been achieved, it is often possible to draw the papilla out into a more favorable position for subsequent manipulations (Figure 3-1B). It is a wise precaution to place a guidewire in the biliary tree or pancreatic duct to maintain position after initial cannulation. This avoids the embarrassment of failing to recannulate after initial success.

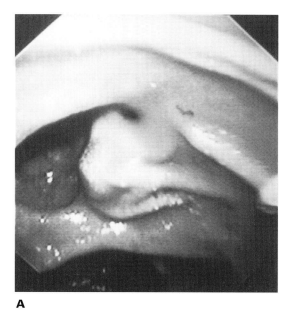

A

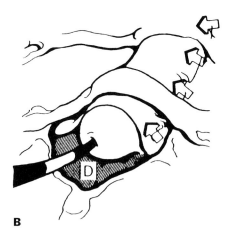

B

Figure 3-1. A. Endoscopic image of papilla within a diverticulum. B. Following deep cannulation, it is often possible to draw the papilla out into a more favorable position for subsequent manipulation. Arrows indicate papillary fold (course of bile duct). (D = diverticulum.)

Sometimes the papilla lies deep within a diverticulum and may be invisible on initial inspection. Blind instrumentation of a diverticulum in the hope of locating an orifice is never justifiable. Poking around diverticula with guidewires and catheters is an invitation to perforation. A useful trick for locating an invisible papilla is to bring the tip of the scope up to the opening of the diverticulum and aspirate air. This procedure sometimes causes the diverticulum to collapse or evert and allows a previously hidden papilla to prolapse into view. Poking the endoscope tip deep into a large diverticulum risks perforation, so this approach should be used with care. If the papilla can be visualized and cannulated by the aspiration technique, it is essential to maintain access using a guidewire. The papilla can often be pulled out into a more favorable position for sphincterotomy or other manipulation once deep cannulation has been achieved.

Another option in case of difficulty is to perform a combined endoscopic-radiologic procedure (combined procedure). First, a wire is placed into the biliary tree by the transcutaneous route at the time of percutaneous transhepatic cholangiography (PTC). Radiologists have become skilled at working in the biliary tree and, once it is accessed, they can often advance a guidewire all the way into the duodenum through the papilla (from

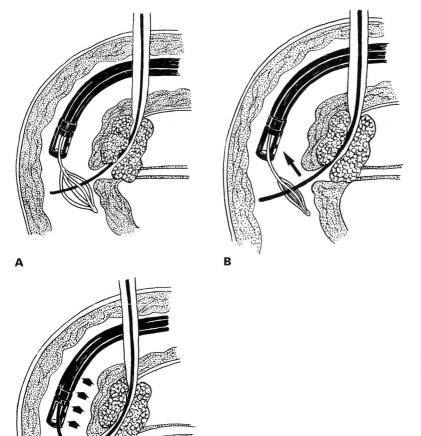

A

B

C

Figure 3-2. Combined procedure. A. Radiologic guidewire advanced into the duodenum from above. B. Once the guidewire is passed into the duodenum, the endoscopist can grasp the wire using a basket catheter. C. Then it is pulled up through the instrument channel of the duodenoscope.

above) (Figure 3-2A). Obviously, there must be a good indication for subjecting any patient to this additional, more invasive procedure. Because PTC is technically difficult when the bile ducts are not dilated, a combined procedure for biliary access should be reserved for patients who have an urgent need for biliary decompression, such as cholangitis or progressive jaundice. Once the guidewire has been passed into the duodenum, the endoscopist can grasp the wire using a basket catheter and pull it up through the instrument channel of the duodenoscope (Figure 3-2B and C). With guidewire access firmly established, endoscopic accessories (e.g., sphincterotomes, stents) can be used in the standard fashion.

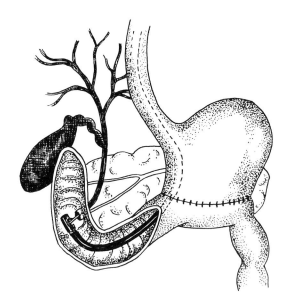

Figure 3-3. Post–Billroth II gastrectomy anatomy.

It is most important that the liver be protected when a guidewire is being used for a combined procedure. At no time should a bare guidewire be pulled through the liver without the protection of some form of oversleeve or catheter. It should not be assumed that the radiologist will automatically understand what you need done during the procedure. Close collaboration is essential; the requirements of the case should be discussed before proceeding. In particular, specific equipment (e.g., a sufficiently long guidewire) should be identified ahead of time.

Postsurgical Anatomy

Surgical diversion of the biliary tree and gastric resection often render ERCP technically difficult. Many endoscopists are reluctant to attempt ERCP in the presence of post–Billroth II (B-II) gastrectomy anatomy. This is a pity, because it is often possible to complete diagnostic and therapeutic ERCP in this situation. The rate-limiting factor is the length of the afferent limb of the gastroenterostomy. If the afferent limb is too long, it is physically impossible for the scope to advance far enough to visualize the duodenal papilla. The B-II reconstruction involves removing the gastric antrum and interrupting the continuity of the duodenum such that there is a blind ending (afferent) limb of the small bowel anastomosis (Figure 3-3). The duodenal papilla lies just a few centimeters distal to the stump of that limb. The technical

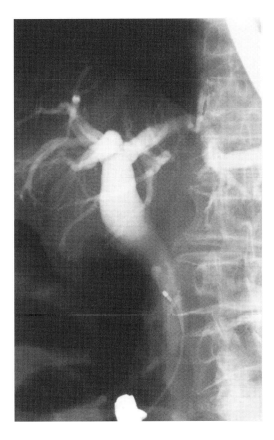

Figure 3-4. Biliary cannulation is often easier from the post–Billroth II approach because it is a relatively straight shot.

problem involved in B-II ERCP is that the normal approach to the papilla is lost. The endoscopic view is, as it were, upside down. The endoscopist needs to have a clear mental picture of the likely orientation of the bile duct and pancreatic duct from this inverted perspective.

Ironically, biliary cannulation is often easier from the B-II approach because it is a relatively straight shot into the bile duct from the B-II scope position (Figure 3-4). Experienced endoscopists find that curved catheters, which are so useful in normal circumstances, are a distinct disadvantage when approaching the papilla from this "wrong" direction. Many of us find that relatively stiff, straight catheters, such as those used for biliary stenting (e.g., inner catheter), are particularly helpful.

Another useful technique is to probe the papillary orifice with the tip of a guidewire to gain access for subsequent catheter placement. My personal preference is to use a hydrophilic or polytetrafluoroethylene- (Teflon) coated guidewire because its softness causes less trauma to the papilla. As always, once deep cannulation has been achieved, the position should be maintained by using a guidewire.

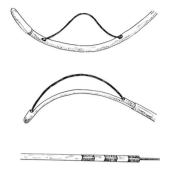

Figure 3-5. A variety of specialized papillotomes.

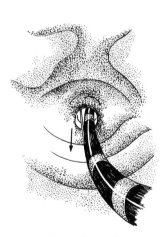

Figure 3-6. The Billroth II sphincterotome has a wire on the bottom of the cannula, which ideally should be oriented in the 6 o'clock position for biliary sphincterotomy. The arrow indicates the desired direction of the cut.

In normal ERCP, the pancreatic duct is frequently the first to be opacified, regardless of the intention of the endoscopist. The situation is reversed in B-II ERCP, where a concerted effort has to be made to find a suitable orientation for pancreatic duct access. This requires advancing the scope beyond the position used for biliary cannulation, to end up in a more en face position. Again, the use of guidewires is invaluable in gaining access and maintaining position. Sometimes it is difficult to access the papilla in the B-II ERCP because of tortuosity of the afferent limb. If this occurs when using a therapeutic duodenoscope (e.g., one with a 4.2-mm instrument channel), it is worth removing the instrument and trying again with a smaller diameter, diagnostic duodenoscope (e.g., 2.8-mm diameter channel). Naturally, this reduces the therapeutic options. If a stent has to be placed with a standard diagnostic duodenoscope, the largest that can be advanced through the instrument channel is 7 Fr.

Endoscopic sphincterotomy of the duodenal papilla is rendered technically more difficult by B-II anatomy. A variety of specialized papillotomes have been developed to address the anatomic considerations (Figure 3-5). Unfortunately, none of these B-II sphincterotomes consistently achieves its promise. The logical design is to have a wire on what would be the bottom of the sphincterotome so that when the cannula is deep in the bile duct the wire is in the 6 o'clock position, ready for cutting (Figure 3-6). In practice, the wire rarely assumes such an accommodating orientation, and considerable manipulation of scope position is needed to achieve the desired axis for the cut. Over the years, I have come to favor using a standard papillotome, which is maneuvered into the required position by endoscopic gymnastics. Usually, a considerable amount of torque (twist) has to be applied to the scope to rotate the tip to allow a normal papillotome to be used. An increasingly popular alternative is needle knife sphincterotomy over a stent.

Needle Knife for Post–Billroth II Sphincterotomy

A technique that works well when a B-II patient requires sphincterotomy is to cut down over a stent using a needle knife. The technique is relatively straightforward. After deep cannulation, a standard plastic endoprosthesis is advanced into the bile duct. The needle knife sphincterotomy is then made by cutting down on top of the stent (Figure 3-7). Provided that the cut is made in the 11 to 1 o'clock arc of safety, it should be relatively safe. Once the sphincterotomy has been performed, the stent may be removed immediately or left for several days to allow edema to settle. If the choice is to remove the stent and proceed with further therapeutic manipulation (usually stone extraction), there are two ways to avoid having to remove the endoscope entirely to recover the stent. If available, a Soehendra-type screw tip extraction device (Wilson-Cook Medical, Inc., Winston-Salem, NC) can be advanced over a wire into the end of the stent (Figure 3-8). The

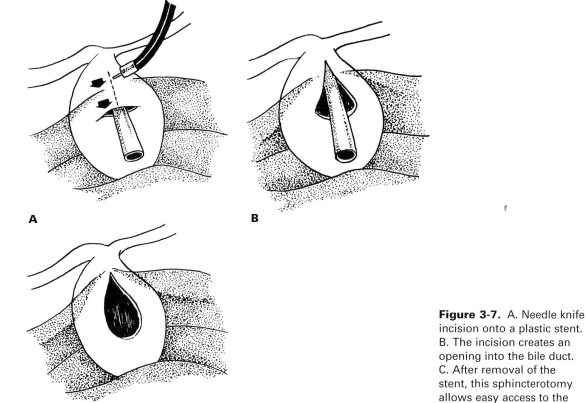

Figure 3-7. A. Needle knife incision onto a plastic stent. B. The incision creates an opening into the bile duct. C. After removal of the stent, this sphincterotomy allows easy access to the biliary tree.

extractor is rotated so that the grooves on the screw tip firmly entrap the stent, which can then be withdrawn through the endoscope channel. At the same time, access to the bile duct is maintained with a guidewire. Another alternative that avoids completely withdrawing the endoscope through the patient's mouth is to remove the stent in the standard fashion using a basket catheter and pull it back into the stomach, where it can be disengaged and left for later retrieval (i.e., on the way out at the end of the procedure).

Roux-en-Y Anastomosis

After partial gastrectomy with a Roux-en-Y type reconstruction, it is rarely possible to gain access to the duodenal papilla using an endoscope. Some endoscopists simply refuse to attempt ERCP in this setting. In expert hands, perhaps only one in five attempts is successful, and therefore it is up

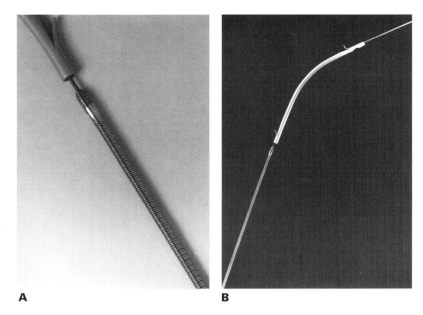

Figure 3-8. A. The screw tip of a stent extraction device. B. Bench demonstration of Soehendra stent extractor. (Courtesy of Wilson-Cook Medical, Inc., Winston-Salem, NC.)

A   **B**

to the individual endoscopist whether or not to attempt ERCP. The alternative is PTC if contrast imaging is essential.

Choledochoduodenostomy

Choledochoduodenostomy (CDD) is the simplest form of biliary bypass procedure. Before the endoscopic era, CDD was sometimes performed for common bile duct stones (choledocholithiasis), especially if the stones were recurrent. With the advent of laparoscopic cholecystectomy (LC), open bile duct exploration has become a rarity, and the use of CDD has declined with it. The usual site of the surgical anastomosis between the gut and the biliary tree is in the posterior duodenal bulb or D1–D2 area (Figure 3-9). A satisfactory CDD should be easily visible to the endoscopist. With time, the opening can progressively shrink, leaving a rather small hole or even a pinhole, which is obviously inadequate for biliary drainage. Although the native papilla is usually left intact, providing another route for endoscopic cannulation, some surgeons transect or otherwise seal off the distal bile duct, rendering standard ERCP cannulation impossible.

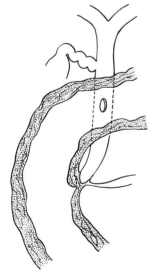

Figure 3-9. The usual site of a surgical choledocho-duodenostomy.

When CDD is performed for presumed papillary stenosis or dysfunction, the length of bile duct distal to the CDD can act as a sump. If its drainage is poor, bacterial overgrowth and stone or sludge formation is likely (Figure 3-10). When patients become symptomatic due to cholangitis or stones in this setting, this is referred to as *sump syndrome*. Where the local anatomy permits, the treatment of sump syndrome is to perform endoscopic sphincterotomy in the standard fashion to improve distal drainage. Due to the rich vasculature of the duodenum, many endoscopists are reluctant to widen the opening of a CDD using electrocautery. A safer alternative is to dilate the opening using a dilating balloon (e.g., Gruntzig type) over a guidewire. Although there are no data on the subject, it is likely that balloon dilatation of a CDD has relatively short-lived benefit. It is certainly possible to place a stent into the biliary tree through a CDD if other means of effecting bile drainage have failed or are unavailable. However, definitive management of a failed CDD requires surgical reconstruction, usually a Roux-en-Y choledochoenterostomy.

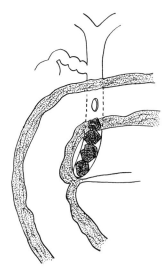

Figure 3-10. Sump syndrome. The excluded distal duct can act as a nidus for infection or stone formation.

Surgical Sphincteroplasty

Surgical enlargement of the bile duct and pancreatic duct orifices is usually an aid to ERCP. Especially if both ducts have been operated on, the orifices are usually separate and obvious. Occasionally, a surgical sphincteroplasty will fibrose down to a narrow opening, and thus, cannulation may become difficult. Due to the fibrous nature of these strictured openings, attempts to widen them by endoscopic sphincterotomy carry an increased risk of complications, such as bleeding and hemorrhage. For this reason, some endoscopists prefer to use balloon dilation on strictured surgical orifices rather than cut them.

Suprapapillary Fistula

The weakest point of the papillary structure is the intraduodenal portion above the papillary orifice. This is the usual site of fistula formation. Suprapapillary fistulae have two causes: (1) surgical or percutaneous passage of guidewires or dilators down the bile duct and (2) spontaneous fistulization by stones. These fistulae rarely cause clinical problems, but they may be the cause of otherwise unexplained pneumobilia. If papillary stenosis is present, the fistula may be the principal (or only) route of bile drainage and access for retrograde cholangiography. If therapeutic access to the bile duct is required, the roof of the papillary fold can be opened by making a cut between the papillary orifice and the fistula (Figure 3-11). This is a relatively safe procedure because the anatomic landmarks are well defined. If the opening produced is inadequate for the purpose, it can be extended cephalad (upward) as room permits. In the occasional patient with severe coagulopathy who needs urgent biliary decompression, a stent or nasobiliary drain can be placed through a suprapapillary fistula as a temporizing maneuver.

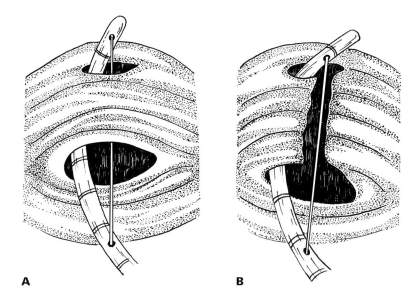

Figure 3-11. A. Before the papillary structure is un-roofed by cutting between the papillary orifice and a suprapapillary fistula. B. After the procedure.

A

B

Papillary Stenosis and Sphincter of Oddi Dysfunction

The flow of bile into the duodenum from the biliary tree is not continuous but intermittent, metered by sphincteric action. The sphincter of Oddi is a smooth muscle valve that encircles the distal common bile duct at the level of the ampulla. The stimuli to sphincter relaxation are not completely understood but are probably a combination of neural, paracrine, and endocrine inputs from the stomach and adjacent duodenum. Papillary stenosis occurs when the sphincteric section of the distal common bile duct becomes fibrosed and narrowed, such that there is obstruction to normal bile flow. The pathophysiology is poorly understood, but one theory often advanced is that the passage of small biliary calculi over time produces a fibrotic reaction.

Stenosis may also result from papillitis in immunocompromised individuals. This ill-defined disorder is presumed to have a viral origin (e.g., cytomegalovirus or human immunodeficiency virus). In classic papillary stenosis, patients have symptoms of biliary colic with abnormal liver function tests (LFTs) and ultrasound evidence of biliary dilatation. These get worse after cholecystectomy, which removes a distensible reservoir (the gallbladder), thereby exacerbating the effect of poor flow into the duodenum. This represents one form of postcholecystectomy pain syndrome. Patients presenting with papillary stenosis have often undergone cholecystectomy for presumed gallstones; it is not unusual for a normal gallbladder to be found at operation. The fibrotic nature of the disorder makes endoscopic cannulation of the bile duct technically difficult in some cases. When

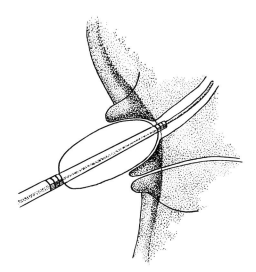

Figure 3-12. Balloon dilatation of the duodenal papilla.

the endoscopic approach fails, consideration should be given to percutaneous access for a combined procedure or referral for surgical sphincteroplasty. Endoscopic sphincterotomy in the presence of papillary stenosis carries an increased risk of complications, such as pancreatitis, bleeding, and perforation. Endoscopic stenting is not a suitable alternative because the risk of pancreatitis is significant. Similarly, balloon dilatation (using a Gruntzig-type dilating balloon) (Figure 3-12) carries significant risk of causing pancreatitis and should be avoided.

Sphincter of Oddi dysfunction (SOD) represents a significant challenge for the ERCP endoscopist. The abnormality is considered a motor disturbance of the sphincter muscle rather than fibrosis, causing episodic symptoms of biliary obstruction and, occasionally, relapsing pancreatitis. Typically, partial obstruction of the biliary tree at the sphincter segment can produce intermittent or persistent upper abdominal pain, elevated LFTs, and distention of the bile duct. Because it is sometimes impossible to distinguish patients with stenosis of the sphincter from those with a motility disorder, Geenen and Hogan have suggested that they be considered together as part of the SOD syndrome. The Geenen-Hogan classification of suspected SOD is represented in Table 3-1 and in the following discussion.

1. Group I patients with suspected SOD present with biliary type pain and elevated LFTs documented on two or more occasions with a dilated bile duct (> 12 mm) or delayed drainage of contrast (> 45 minutes) from the common bile duct during ERCP. Using biliary manometry, motor dysfunction has been recorded in 65–70% of these patients. Sphincter of Oddi stenosis appears to predominate in this group. Endoscopic sphincterotomy

Table 3-1. Modified Geenen-Hogan classification of sphincter of Oddi dysfunction (excludes delayed drainage)

Geenen-Hogan class	Pain	Abnormal liver function tests on two occasions	Dilated common bile duct ≧ 12 mm in diameter
I	Yes	Yes	Yes
II	Yes	Yes	No
	Yes	No	Yes
III	Yes	No	No

in group I patients almost always abolishes their symptoms, confirming that some partial obstruction of the distal bile duct is the etiology of the problem. Because the results of sphincterotomy are so favorable in this group of patients, prior manometry is considered unnecessary.

2. Group II patients have biliary type pain but only one of the two other criteria listed for group I. Sphincter of Oddi motor dysfunction occurs in half of this group. In group II patients, the prevalence of a motility disorder (dyskinesia) and stenosis appear to be similar.

3. Group III patients with suspected SOD present clinically with a pain syndrome only. Sphincter of Oddi manometry is abnormal in less than 10% of group III patients. In group III patients who have abnormal manometry findings, only half improve following endoscopic sphincterotomy.

For the gastroenterologist who sees patients with pancreatic and biliary disorders, SOD is one of the most difficult management problems. Patients referred for ERCP to evaluate "biliary" pain have often undergone extensive radiologic investigation without benefit. Unfortunately, chronic right upper quadrant abdominal pain may arise from a large number of sources, ranging from pleurisy and chest wall fibromyalgia to urosepsis and spastic colon. Provocative tests of biliary pain that rely on drug administration or balloon distention of the bile duct do not correlate with objective measurements of biliary motor dysfunction. As Hogan has pointed out, abdominal pain is the apparent clinical manifestation of most functional GI disorders. Before undertaking aggressive treatment for presumed papillary stenosis or SOD, some causal relationship must be established between the dysfunction and the pain. Patients with "biliary dyskinesia" are frequently found to have other functional GI problems, including esophageal dysmotility, gastroesophageal reflux disorder, and irritable bowel syndrome. Such patients may have heightened awareness of visceral distention and motility. This syndrome has been dubbed *heightened visceral nociception*.

Since its promulgation in the late 1980s, the Geenen-Hogan classification has served as a useful guide to those of us who look after patients with biliary-type pain. Recently, the observation that there are patients with no demonstrable evidence of sphincter stenosis or papillary dyskinesia who clearly benefit from endoscopic sphincterotomy has stimulated a reevaluation of the Geenen-Hogan classification, particularly as it relates to group III patients. In particular, the concept of biliary manometry as a gold standard has been questioned. Other techniques, including radionuclide biliary emptying studies (e.g., CCK-HIDA cholescintigraphy) and biliary ultrasound before and after fatty meal stimulation have been offered as alternatives to manometry before deciding on endoscopic or surgical therapy.

Bile Duct Calculi (Choledocholithiasis)

One of the most successful applications of therapeutic ERCP has been in the management of stones in the biliary tree. Choledocholithiasis can and often does occur in the absence of a gallbladder (i.e., postcholecystectomy). The common problems associated with stones in the bile duct are pain, infection (cholangitis), acute or intermittent biliary obstruction, and pancreatitis. Acute cholangitis is a medical emergency and an indication for urgent biliary decompression by either endoscopic or percutaneous drainage. It should be remembered that cholangitis carries significant mortality when treatment is delayed. The minimum therapeutic skill that any ERCP endoscopist should have is the ability to ensure adequate biliary drainage. When it is difficult or impossible to completely remove stones or other obstructions causing cholangitis in the bile duct, a stent or nasobiliary drain must be left at the end of the procedure. If this proves impossible, the endoscopist has a duty to ensure that the patient is sent for urgent percutaneous biliary drainage or, where necessary, surgery.

Why stones form in the biliary tree is not entirely clear, but it is presumably a combination of factors. Some patients have lithogenic bile, that is, they tend to precipitate cholesterol out of solution to form sludge, gravel, and finally stones. Patients with periampullary diverticula are at increased risk of developing bile duct stones. It is thought that diverticula provide foci for bacterial overgrowth and ascending infection through the papilla into the bile duct. In addition, diverticula may interfere in some way with normal sphincter of Oddi motility.

Foreign bodies of various kinds are well known to act as nidi for stone formation. Surgical sutures and clips are especially common in bile duct stones (Figure 3-13). In parts of the world where biliary infestation with liver flukes is endemic (e.g., Southeast Asia), choledocholithiasis is extremely common. The ova of liver flukes, such as *Clonorchis sinensis* and *Fasciola hepatica*, and the bodies of dead adult worms, often can be identified in sections of bile duct stones. Although pure cholesterol stones are encountered, the predominant bile duct stone is a mixture of pigment (calcium bilirubinate) and cholesterol held together in an organic matrix

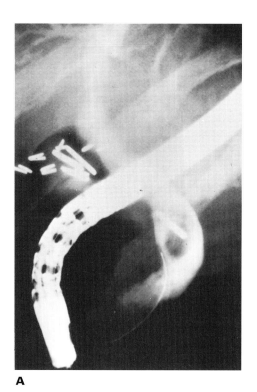

A

Figure 3-13. Bile duct stones often grow around surgical sutures and clips. A. Cholangiogram shows that the stone in the bile duct contains a linear opacity (cat's eye sign). B. When the stone is removed using a basket catheter, the opacity is seen to be a metallic surgical clip.

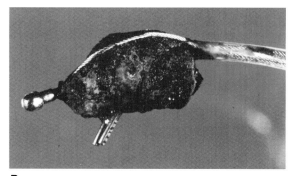

B

(brown pigment stones). Depending on the ratio of pigment to cholesterol, the stones may become extremely hard, resisting mechanical and other forms of lithotripsy. Patients with chronic hemolysis are predisposed to develop pure pigment stones secondary to excessive hemoglobin breakdown and hepatic excretion.

Common Bile Duct Stone Removal

Since its introduction in 1974, endoscopic sphincterotomy has become the standard way to enter the extrahepatic bile duct for stone extraction. It has recently been demonstrated, however, that small stones can be recovered without sphincterotomy using balloon and basket catheters. Firm traction on the stone allows it to be pulled through the intact papilla. The first report of a series of patients treated this way came from Duke University. We saw surprisingly few complications. Balloon dilatation of the papilla was used in several patients to facilitate access, but in most cases (especially when the stone is < 5 mm) this is unnecessary. A group from Ireland subsequently reported the use of balloon dilatation to allow quite large stones (10–15 mm) to be removed from the common bile duct without sphincterotomy. It surprised many of us that such impressive dilatation of the papilla seemed to be tolerated without complications. Data from studies using this approach are still being collated, but in expert hands it seems to work.

Stone extraction without sphincterotomy is attractive because it avoids the risks and late complications (e.g., stenosis, stone re-formation) of sphincterotomy. This approach gives us another management option in young patients with choledocholithiasis, in whom we wish to avoid sphincter ablation. However, there will be no dramatic reduction in the use of endoscopic sphincterotomy in the foreseeable future. Following an adequate sphincterotomy, small stones can usually be cleared from the bile duct using a retrieval balloon, basket catheter, or a combination of both. If the stones are soft, they crumble into a watery paste as they are being removed. At the end of a long procedure when multiple stones like this have been crushed, a great deal of putty-like debris may remain in the bile duct. It is a wise precaution after such procedures to place a stent or nasobiliary drain to ensure that a plug of debris does not occlude the sphincterotomy orifice. In one case we encountered at Duke University, there were so many stones in the biliary tree that many remained after three attempts to clear them (Figure 3-14). The eventual solution was forcibly lavaging the remaining stones out of the bile duct using the pressure wash capacity of an endoscopic heater probe that was advanced well into the hilum.

Dissolution Therapy

In the past, we tried to dissolve large bile duct stones using cholesterol-dissolving agents (e.g., mono-octanoin) infused through a nasobiliary drain, but the technique was slow, cumbersome, and limited by frequent side effects. With modern endoscopic techniques, it is now a rarity to be defeated by common bile duct stones and so dissolution methods have fallen out

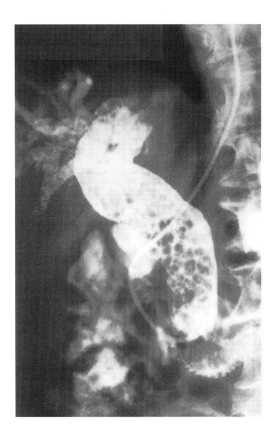

Figure 3-14. Nasobiliary cholangiogram showing massive distention of the biliary tree with small calculi.

of favor. Methyl tert-butyl ether, which has been used with success for gall-stone dissolution in the gallbladder, is unsuitable for use in the bile duct because of containment problems. What we require is a solvent that consistently disaggregates mixed bile duct stones and has few if any toxic side effects or safety problems. At present, none has been identified.

Mechanical Lithotripsy

Large, soft stones may be crushed into smaller pieces using endoscopic baskets. Care should be taken not to entrap a stone in a basket if that stone cannot be crushed or subsequently disengaged. In the old days, basket impaction during attempted stone extraction often led to the operating room. Although it is still an unpleasant occurrence, entrapment of a stone in a basket is no longer such a problem. We deal with this as follows: The handle of the basket is removed and the endoscope withdrawn over the basket catheter, leaving the end exiting from the patient's mouth.

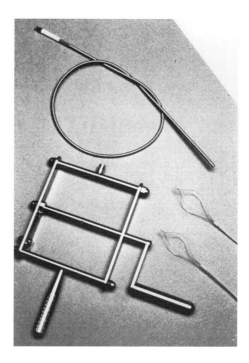

Figure 3-15. Tools of mechanical lithotripsy. When a basket catheter (lower right) gets trapped in the bile duct, the mechanical crank (lower left) can save the day. The handle of the catheter is removed and the oversleeve (top) is advanced down its shaft until it is snug against the entrapped stone. The wires of the snare (exposed after the handle is removed) are threaded through the opening in the metal crank and wound around the central spindle. When the handle is cranked, the wires are tightened, causing either the stone or the basket to break.

A flexible metal oversleeve is then passed over the basket catheter until the end abuts the wires holding the stone. The free end of the basket catheter is then stripped to expose bare wires, which are wound around the cranking device. The end of the cranking device fits onto the upper end of the metal sleeve. When the crank is wound tight, the wires of the snare are pulled forcibly against the metal sleeve (Figure 3-15). One of two things happens: Either the stone or the wires break, but in either case it takes care of the problem.

What constitutes a large stone? Most authors agree that bile duct stones exceeding 15 mm in diameter present a challenge to remove because it is difficult to make the orifice of a sphincterotomy any larger than this. When standard balloon or basket retrieval fails, large mechanical lithotriptors can be used to apply enormous forces to break up stones. These are so effective that other forms of lithotripsy (e.g., laser, electrohydraulic, percutaneous) are now almost obsolete.

Intrahepatic stones present a particular problem for the endoscopist because they are so hard to reach. It is rarely possible to completely clear an intrahepatic biliary tree of multiple stones, particularly if strictures are present (e.g., as in primary sclerosing cholangitis). A percutaneous approach may be preferable for some patients, and surgery may ultimately be needed to decompress chronically obstructed ducts or resect affected liver segments or lobes.

Contact Lithotripsy

Direct contact lithotripsy using a laser beam requires a specialized type of laser that delivers pulsed rather than continuous energy. For example, the Candela tunable dye laser (Candela, Boston, MA) operates at a frequency of about 10 Hz. Each pulse of laser energy causes vaporization at the surface of the stone, resulting in a shock wave that propagates fissures throughout the material. Electrohydraulic lithotripsy is another, less expensive, variation on the same theme. Contact lithotripsy in the bile duct is often successful. Laser lithotripsy, however, is expensive and time consuming, making it a technique that only a few large centers can afford. Automatic stone detection systems may render laser lithotripsy more accurate and less likely to cause collateral drainage.

When contact methods for stone fragmentation are unavailable or fail, extrahepatic shock wave lithotripsy (ESWL) is a viable alternative. Contrast injected through a nasobiliary drain provides necessary targeting information and allows the progress of the procedure to be monitored fluoroscopically. Although stone fragments created by ESWL can be lavaged out of the bile duct using the nasobiliary drain, a further ERCP is usually required to clear the biliary tree completely.

Mirizzi Syndrome

Gallstones that lodge in the cystic duct or Hartmann's pouch of the gallbladder can cause extrahepatic biliary obstruction by direct pressure on the common bile duct or common hepatic duct, depending on the site of insertion of the cystic duct. The often smooth, extrinsic compression mimics a malignant stricture (Figure 3-16), but ultrasound or computed tomographic (CT) scanning can usually reveal the true nature of the problem. Endoscopic biliary stenting usually provides excellent palliation in this situation. In fit patients, surgery is the definitive treatment. For patients considered unfit for surgery, ESWL may be an alternative, although if the stone is entrapped in a fibrotic cavity, ESWL simply turns the stone into powder, which will remain in the same place. Percutaneous access can be used to reach the offending stone for contact lithotripsy and fragment removal.

Stents for Bile Duct Stones

An option when bile duct stones defy extraction—before or after various forms of lithotripsy—is to leave one or more stents in the bile duct. These ensure biliary drainage and may reduce the size of the residual stone or stones by encouraging fragmentation. It is often possible to clear the biliary tree of stones when follow-up ERCP is performed after a suitable interval

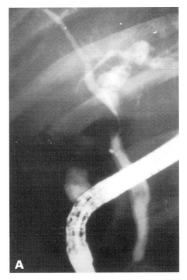

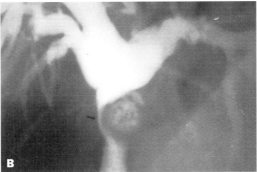

Figure 3-16. Mirizzi syndrome. A. A stone in the cystic duct or Hartmann's pouch can mimic a malignant stricture, in this case of the common hepatic duct. B. The cystic duct stone lying to the left of the obstructed common hepatic duct is partially calcified, revealing the diagnosis.

to retrieve or exchange the stent. The use of ursodeoxycholate therapy to accelerate stone dissolution may be a useful adjunct to stenting.

Surgery for Bile Duct Stones

Surgery is not the worst fate that can befall a patient with retained bile duct stones. In cases where stones have resisted the usual endoscopic or percutaneous approaches, consideration should be given to surgery. An open common bile duct exploration with a drainage procedure may be less traumatic to the patient than several less invasive but unsuccessful procedures. Elderly patients with or without significant comorbidities are often deemed unfit for surgery by nonsurgeons. Before making such a pronouncement, however, formal evaluation of the patient by an experienced biliary surgeon

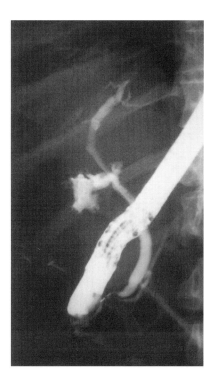

Figure 3-17. Cholangiogram showing extravasation of contrast at the level of the cystic duct stump in a patient with a postcholecystectomy bile duct leak.

and an anesthesiologist is appropriate. Many elderly patients sail through bile duct surgery without incident.

Bile Duct Leaks

Bile leakage most commonly follows gallbladder surgery, when failure to completely clip off the cystic duct, injury to the common bile duct or common hepatic duct, or inadvertent rupture of aberrant hepatic ducts draining into the gallbladder result in extravasation of bile into potential spaces around the liver (Figure 3-17). A walled-off collection of bile is often referred to as a *biloma*. Following orthotopic liver transplantation, breakdown of the surgical anastomosis or failure of the T-tube track to close may result in a biloma. Bile duct leaks are seen occasionally following percutaneous liver biopsy and penetrating trauma. Appropriate management requires prompt identification of the leak site. Increasingly, the radioisotope HIDA scan is used to confirm the presence of a leak. This test is noninvasive but purely diagnostic; ERCP is both diagnostic and therapeutic. If the leak site remains open, contrast injected for cholangiography will demonstrate the abnormality by extravasation.

The majority of bile leaks can be managed by one or more of the following techniques: stent placement, nasobiliary drainage, or sphincterotomy. Unless there is mechanical obstruction to bile flow (such as an impacted stone or papillary stenosis) that would clearly benefit from sphincterotomy, the procedure is unnecessary and its attendant risks unjustifiable. Nasobiliary drainage often results in closure of a leak within a few days. If a nasobiliary drain is used, it should be placed on low wall suction for maximum benefit. Endoscopic stents reduce the pressure gradient across the papilla and encourage distal flow of bile (i.e., away from the leak) (Figure 3-18). There is considerable debate about how long the stent should be. Many endoscopists prefer to place a stent with its proximal end above the level of the leak, in the hope that in some way this seals off the offending area, but similar results can be achieved with short stents straddling the papilla.

Because most biliary leaks seal off within days after endoscopic therapy, there is little point in leaving stents or drains in place for many weeks or months. Therefore, stents should be removed after 2–4 weeks. Repeat ERCP for stent removal may be rendered unnecessary in the near future by the introduction of biodegradable stents. Bilomas large enough to be targeted by ultrasound or CT imaging should be drained because they may become infected or rupture into the peritoneum or pleural cavity, causing serious complications.

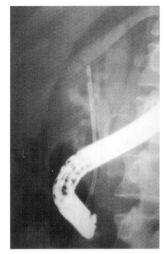

Figure 3-18. An endoscopic biliary stent placed to correct a leak.

Biliary Strictures

Biliary tract strictures may be intrahepatic or extrahepatic, benign or malignant. The most common benign strictures ERCP endoscopists encounter are due to surgical injury (especially after LC), chronic pancreatitis, sclerosing cholangitis, and (in specialist centers) those related to liver transplantation. The most common malignancies causing biliary strictures are carcinoma of the pancreas, bile duct cancers (cholangiocarcinoma), gallbladder carcinoma, and a variety of metastatic malignancies (e.g., lung, breast, colon). Primary liver cancers (hepatoma) usually cause their LFT abnormalities and symptoms by compression of parenchyma and less often by direct pressure on the biliary tree. Certain stricturing conditions have a typical appearance. In sclerosing cholangitis, for example, a chronic fibrotic process usually associated with inflammatory bowel disease, there can be strictures in the intrahepatic and extrahepatic biliary tree (Figure 3-19). Few conditions mimic sclerosing cholangitis, but diagnostic difficulty may occur when there is a single, dominant extrahepatic stricture. Given that the sensitivity of cytologic and biopsy techniques in the biliary tree is considerably less than 100%, a definitive diagnosis may require surgical exploration and resection.

Distinguishing between benign and malignant biliary strictures is extremely important in determining their subsequent management. Cytologic

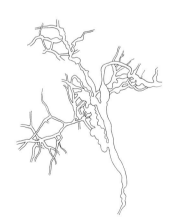

Figure 3-19. Schematic from cholangiogram showing primary sclerosing cholangitis with characteristic bile duct strictures.

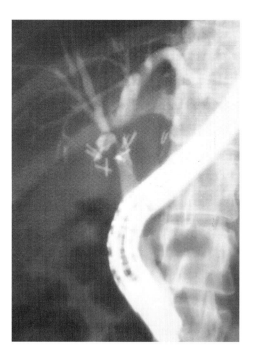

Figure 3-20. Cholangiogram showing a hilar bile duct stricture caused by misplaced surgical clips (postlaparoscopic cholecystectomy bile duct injury).

brushing is the most direct and easily applied technique. Postsurgical strictures, as are seen after thermal or mechanical injury at cholecystectomy, and those seen after liver transplantation, are rarely difficult to diagnose (Figure 3-20). In transplant patients, the strictures are usually anastomotic (Figure 3-21). Postcholecystectomy strictures are often short and localized to the region of the cystic duct origin. By contrast, malignant strictures are often long, with irregular or *shouldered* margins (Figure 3-22). Malignant strictures causing obstructive jaundice often cause marked proximal dilatation of the bile ducts (Figure 3-23). Carcinoma at the head of the pancreas typically involves both the common bile duct as it passes through the head of the pancreas and the main pancreatic duct, resulting in the double duct sign (Figure 3-24).

Endoscopic biliary stenting is frequently used to palliate malignant strictures and to provide initial therapy for benign strictures. The latter are generally unsuitable for long-term stenting in younger patients, who probably require definitive surgery. As a rule, we use dilating balloons or graduated dilators to stretch benign biliary strictures before placing stents. How long should a patient with a benign bile duct stricture undergo repeated balloon dilatation and stenting before surgery is performed? There are limited data on the subject, but our preference at Duke University is to stent the asymptomatic patient for up to 1 year (or a total of three stents) before referring

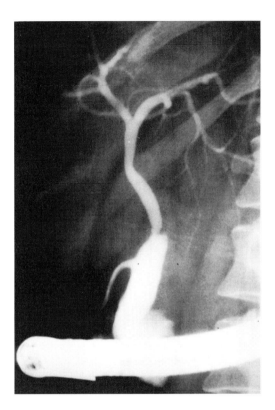

Figure 3-21. Bile duct strictures in liver transplant patients usually occur at the anastomosis. This cholangiogram also demonstrates a persistent leak at the T-tube site, a not infrequent problem after transplantation.

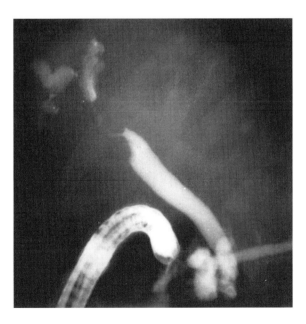

Figure 3-22. Cholangiogram showing a malignant hilar bile duct stricture.

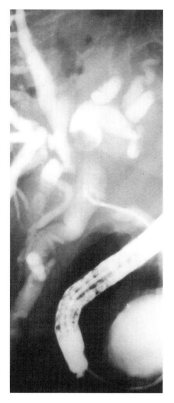

Figure 3-23. Gross proximal dilatation of the biliary tree above a malignant stricture.

him or her for surgery if the stricture is unchanged. With rare exceptions, we have avoided using expandable metal mesh stents to treat benign biliary strictures. When further generations of these stents become easily exchangeable, we will have less concern about the long-term implications of placing what is essentially a permanent device in the biliary tree.

The easiest strictures to treat are low in the bile duct. Short, soft, head of pancreas tumors provide an ideal training ground for ERCP novices. Many benign strictures are firm and resist access with standard guidewires and catheters. Hydrophilic or Teflon-coated guidewires are particularly useful when tight strictures provide this kind of challenge. Hilar strictures appear in three levels of difficulty (Figure 3-25).

1. Type I hilar strictures involve the common hepatic duct up to but not including the bifurcation. If a stent can be advanced just through the stricture, both sides of the liver should be decompressed.

2. Type II hilar strictures include the bifurcation. In these strictures, decompression has to be provided separately for each side of the liver. This requires two stents or percutaneous drains if endoscopic access proves impossible.

3. Type III biliary strictures involve the duct beyond the hilum and cause obstruction of multiple segments. Palliation of these tumors represents a significant challenge because several segments of the liver may have to be decompressed. When a liver tumor grows so large that much of the parenchyma is involved, it becomes impossible for the bile ducts to dilate. In these cases, jaundice, itching, and grossly abnormal LFTs cannot be palliated using biliary stents or drains. Cross-sectional imaging (ultrasound, CT scanning) prior to attempting biliary decompression is important in such patients because the absence of obvious dilated biliary radicals is a contraindication to the procedure.

Sclerosing Cholangitis

Sclerosing cholangitis is the term applied to a large spectrum of pathologic processes that results in bile duct injury. The abnormalities seen include inflammation, fibrosis, thickening of the bile duct wall, and stricture formation. Primary sclerosing cholangitis (PSC) is that not clearly associated with other causes (Table 3-2).

Patients with PSC may be suspected of having this diagnosis when they are referred for ERCP. They have often already had a liver biopsy to investigate abnormal LFTs (with or without jaundice). By this time, the hepatologist has eliminated the usual viral and autoimmune hepatitides, as well as drug reaction, from the differential diagnosis. Cross-sectional abdominal imaging usually shows no biliary abnormality. In more advanced cases, however, segmental bile duct dilation with stone formation may be demonstrated. The way PSC presents depends on the nature of the disease process.

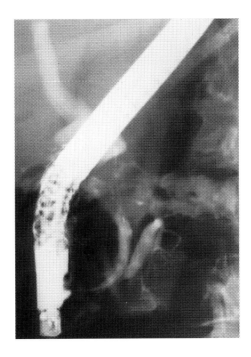

Figure 3-24. The classic double duct sign of pancreatic carcinoma.

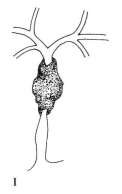 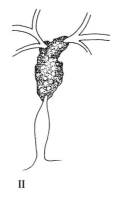 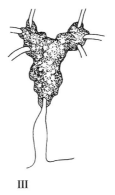

I   II   III

Figure 3-25. The three types of biliary hilar strictures. Type I. Stricture is below and does not involve bifurcation. Type II. Stricture involves bifurcation and extends up into the main hepatic ducts. Type III. Complex hilar stricture involves major and minor intrahepatic ducts.

Patients with a single, dominant extrahepatic bile duct stricture may develop progressive jaundice, pruritus, cholangitis, or all three. If the stricture has been present for long enough, stones may form above it. Intrahepatic bile duct involvement often starts as a quite subtle process. Indeed, the patient may be asymptomatic and the problem only comes to light because of the incidental finding of deranged LFTs. Liver biopsy may show small bile duct changes suggestive of a chronic inflammatory process, such as pericholangitis, or, often, more nonspecific abnormalities. Rarely, patients present with chronic liver injury resulting in cirrhosis and portal hyperten-

Table 3-2. Classification of sclerosing cholangitis

Primary
    Unknown cause associated with other diseases (e.g., ulcerative colitis)
Secondary
    Known or suspected causes
        Surgical trauma
        Bile duct stones
        Cholangiocarcinoma
        Toxic agents (e.g., formaldehyde)
        Ischemia
        Intrahepatic arterial floxuridine (and derivatives)
        Transplant rejection
        Histocytosis X
        Acquired immunodeficiency syndrome (*Cryptosporidium* infection)

Source: Adapted from SC Lu, N Kaplowitz. Diseases of the Biliary Tree. In T Yamada, et al. (eds), Textbook of Gastroenterology. Philadelphia: Lippincott, 1991;1990.

sion. Those who have chronic biliary sepsis complicating PSC may develop liver abscesses.

What can the endoscopist contribute to the management of PSC patients? First, ERCP usually confirms the diagnosis. Figure 3-26 shows typical PSC appearance at three levels, ranging from subtle to gross. Second, there may be an opportunity to attempt endoscopic therapy. Although therapeutic ERCP has nothing to offer PSC patients with extensive intrahepatic disease (multiple structures of segmental and subsegmental ducts), dominant extrahepatic strictures may be dilated and stented repeatedly to improve biliary drainage. Small stones above a dominant biliary stricture may be removed after endoscopic dilatation. It is important to appreciate, however, that therapeutic ERCP does not prevent the progression of PSC; it simply palliates obstruction. Repeated endoscopic retrograde cholangiography or ERCP to follow the progress of PSC in an otherwise well patient cannot be justified and puts the patient at risk from endoscopically introduced infection. Because the most severely affected PSC patients are now referred for liver transplantation, it is important to avoid surgical procedures, such as biliary diversion, that interfere with the transplant process. For this reason, therapeutic ERCP has become an important adjunct in the management of severe PSC, keeping symptoms, such as pruritus, and complications, such as cholangitis, in check until the patient can receive a new liver.

The ERCP endoscopist should be aware that PSC predisposes the biliary tree to malignant change. Accessible strictures should be brushed for cytology and biopsied whenever possible to look for evidence of cholangiocarcinoma. Bile duct dilation proximal to a dominant PSC stricture is unusual. Fibrosis of the bile duct wall makes it less distensible than normal. When

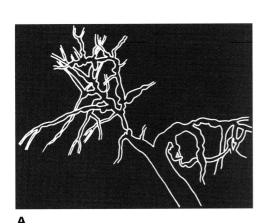

A

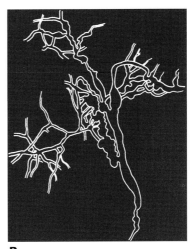

B

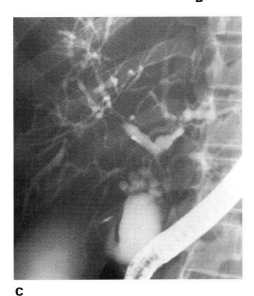

C

Figure 3-26. Stages of sclerosing cholangitis. A. Primary sclerosing cholangitis confined to intraheptic ducts. This schematic is a tracing of an actual cholangiogram. Note the subtle stricturing and focally dilated ducts. B. Primary sclerosing cholangitis involving both intrahepatic and extrahepatic ducts (tracing from an actual cholangiogram). The solitary extraheptic (common bile duct) stricture may respond to endoscopic therapy. C. Advanced primary sclerosing cholangitis with gross ductal abnormalities.

significant dilation of the bile duct is seen above a stricture, especially if the patient becomes unwell after a long period of stability, malignancy should be suspected. In addition to cytology, flow cytometry and tumor markers may be helpful in identifying malignant change in PSC strictures. When the endoscopic approach to PSC strictures fails, skilled vascular (interventional) radiologists can often provide percutaneous access for further manipulations, including combined endoscopic-radiologic procedures. Of interest, a syndrome almost indistinguishable from PSC has been seen in AIDS patients. This *AIDS cholangiopathy* occurs in association with fungal and viral infection of the biliary tree (*Cryptosporidium*, cytomegalovirus). An apparent papillitis, causing sphincter of Oddi stenosis, may be seen in the same patients.

Endoscopic Retrograde Cholangiopancreatography in Relation to Laparoscopic Cholecystectomy

A great deal has been written and said about the role of ERCP before and after LC. This minimally invasive procedure is now the standard approach to removing the gallbladder. When it was first introduced, endoscopists saw many bile duct injuries and leaks, which reflected the surgeons' learning curve. Fortunately, we now see far fewer problems of this nature, although specialist centers are still asked to help with complications on a regular basis. The discussion of ERCP in relation to LC can be divided into (1) the management of bile duct stones and (2) the management of complications (leaks, strictures).

Management of Common Bile Duct Stones

The ERCP endoscopist is frequently asked to perform ERCP before or after LC because of the suspicion of bile duct stones on ultrasound scanning, radionuclide studies (e.g., HIDA), or intravenous or intraoperative cholangiography. The algorithm for the use of diagnostic and therapeutic ERCP depends on the operative technique (does the surgeon routinely perform intraoperative cholangiography or choledochoscopy?), the skill and experience of the endoscopist, and the indication for the procedure (Figure 3-27). If the endoscopist is skilled and has a high success rate for bile duct cannulation (> 90%), the surgeon may await the outcome of intraoperative cholangiography during LC in cases where a bile duct stone is suspected (i.e., the ERCP is performed after LC only if an abnormality is found). If, on the other hand, the surgeon does not have skilled endoscopic support, he or she may request preoperative ERCP. If biliary cannulation fails, the surgeon then has the option of performing open cholecystectomy with bile duct exploration should a stone be found, referring the patient postoperatively to a more experienced endoscopist for another attempt at ERCP, or engaging the services of a skilled interventional radiologist for percutaneous access to the biliary tree.

In terms of risk of choledocholithiasis, patients can be divided into high-risk (> 20%) and low-risk (< 5%) categories according to imaging and serologic tests. Patients with obstructive jaundice, cholangitis, and apparent stones on ultrasound imaging are likely to have stones at ERCP. Many surgeons prefer to have the biliary tree decompressed endoscopically before LC in such cases, to reduce the risk of septic and renal problems after surgery.

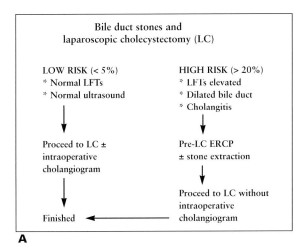

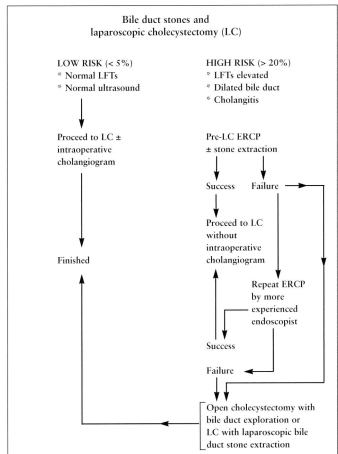

Figure 3-27. A. Algorithm for management of common bile duct stones in patients undergoing laparoscopic cholecystectomy (LC), stratified by risk. Those at intermediate risk probably do not require pre-LC endoscopic retrograde cholangiopancreatography (ERCP). B. Algorithm for management of common bile duct stones in patients undergoing LC. Failed ERCP prior to LC may be managed by repeat ERCP by a more experienced endoscopist, or the surgeon may choose open cholecystectomy with common bile duct exploration or laparoscopic bile duct stone extraction as alternatives. (LFTs = liver function tests.)

It is helpful for the endoscopist to leave a nasobiliary drain in the bile duct to facilitate intraoperative cholangiography at LC if large stones have been removed and debris left. If pre-LC ERCP for duct clearance is performed, it is wise for the patient to proceed to LC without undue delay. An interval of weeks or longer can allow stones to pass from the gallbladder or cystic duct into the common bile duct, negating the benefit of the prior ERCP. In the early days of LC, intraoperative ERCP had its advocates, but these combined endoscopic-laparoscopic adventures significantly prolong operating room time and are not always successful. It is now customary to perform ERCP and LC on separate days. Because ERCP in LC patients may be technically challenging (they often have normal-caliber ducts that are difficult to reach), it should only be performed if there is a good indication to do so. Consideration should be given to removing small stones found at ERCP by techniques that avoid sphincterotomy (see previous discussion under Common Bile Duct Stone Removal). This avoids the need for sphincter ablation, which is particularly undesirable in young adults.

Management of Bile Duct Injuries

The majority of bile duct leaks following LC can be dealt with by placing an endoscopic stent with the distal end in the duodenum (Figure 3-28). Although some experts routinely perform endoscopic sphincterotomy, others believe that it is overkill unless there is a mechanical obstruction to bile outflow, such as an impacted stone or true papillary stenosis.

Considerable debate surrounds the optimum length and size (circumference, in French scale) of the stent used. There are no good data to suggest that long stents (i.e., those that cover the site of the leak) are more effective than short ones (i.e., those that simply bridge the duodenal papilla). Similarly, there is no proof that 10 Fr stents are better than 7 Fr, or that multiple stents are better than single ones. Clearly, a variety of interventions achieve the same end result: The vast majority of the leaks close. Stents should be removed after 2–4 weeks. In the future, these cases will be eminently suitable for the use of biodegradable stents that self-destruct in a predictable fashion, thus avoiding the need for a second endoscopic procedure. Such stents are currently in development.

Why do a few bile leaks persist despite stenting? Sometimes, the stent migrates, thereby adding to the problem. In other cases, the leak site may be so large that stenting alone is insufficient. Sometimes, nasobiliary drainage to low wall suction allows the fistula to heal, but this necessitates in-patient admission and the use of a nasobiliary drain, which patients find uncomfortable. Leaks from transected bile ducts supplying liver segments VI–VIII seem particularly prone to persist despite endoscopic intervention (Figure 3-29). It is sometimes necessary to perform percutaneous cholangiography to reach the injured duct and establish percutaneous drainage. Almost always, these injuries require formal surgical repair (usually a Roux-en-Y choledochojejunostomy). Localizing the source of difficult leaks

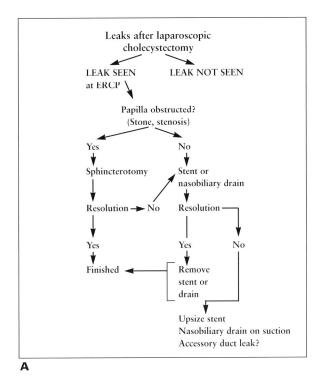

A

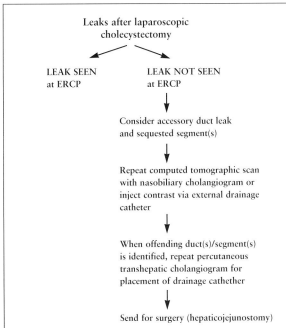

B

Figure 3-28. A. Algorithm for management of biliary leaks after laparoscopic cholecystectomy if the leak is seen during cholangiography. B. Algorithm for management of biliary leaks after laparoscopic cholecystectomy if the leak is not seen on cholangiography. (ERCP = endoscopic retrograde cholangiopancreatography.)

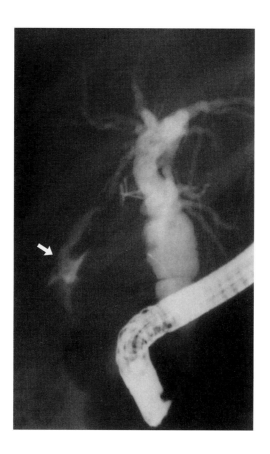

Figure 3-29. Bile duct leak due to an accessory duct (arrow). Such leaks may fail to respond to endoscopic intervention, such as stenting or sphincterotomy.

is facilitated by taking late ERCP films; a small pool of extravasated contrast may appear late in a series of cholangiograms. All films should be developed and studied closely before the duodenoscope is removed and the ERCP considered complete.

Strictures of the bile duct may develop early or late due to thermal or mechanical injury (e.g., from clips partially or wholly across the duct). Complete ductal occlusion or transection is not remediable by therapeutic endoscopy (Figure 3-30). Typically, patients present within 3–7 days of surgery with malaise and progressive jaundice. The site of injury is often defined better by PTC than by ERCP, and percutaneous biliary drainage needs to be established pending surgical reconstruction. Incomplete strictures may be dilated and stented in an effort to avoid surgery. The decision to refer a patient for reconstructive surgery depends on symptoms, LFT results (normal or abnormal), and response to nonsurgical therapy (dilatation or stenting). Because there are often medicolegal issues (threat of litigation), these decisions have to be made carefully, preferably by a multidisciplinary team with expertise in managing hepatobiliary disorders. Sequestration of segmental bile ducts may be missed unless particular

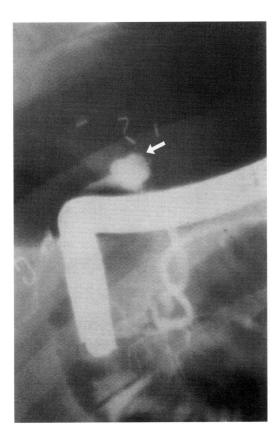

Figure 3-30. Complete transection of the bile duct (arrow). This severe injury inevitably requires surgical repair. It is not amenable to endoscopic therapy.

attention is devoted to full opacification of the intrahepatic biliary tree. Failure of the right lobe to opacify due to occlusion of the right main hepatic duct may be missed if the ductopenia is not appreciated (Figure 3-31). Again, PTC may be required to opacify the sequestered system and effect drainage prior to definitive surgical repair (Figure 3-32).

It is a common finding at surgery that the ductal injury is more extensive than suggested by the cholangiography. This is especially true for ischemic (vascular) injuries. Progressive extension of an ischemic stricture can and does result in occlusion of surgical diversions that are created too close to the injury site.

Choledochal Cysts

Cystic dilatation of the biliary tree is a congenital abnormality that may be localized or diffuse. Choledochal cysts range from a short, fusiform dilatation (Figure 3-33A) to a long, saccular one that may involve the entire

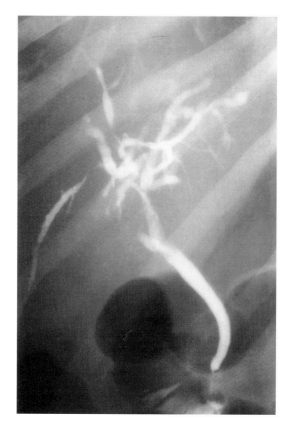

Figure 3-31. Much of the right side of the liver is not seen on this cholangiogram. Failure to appreciate that some or all of the right main hepatic duct branches are missing on a cholangiogram may result in a missed diagnosis.

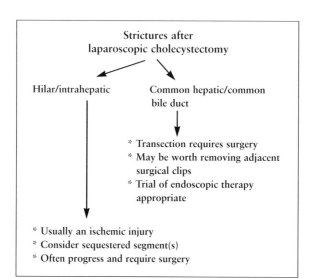

Figure 3-32. Algorithm for managing post–laparoscopic cholecystectomy bile duct stricture.

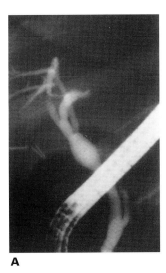

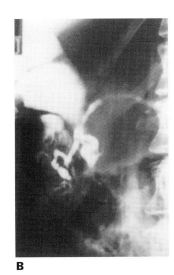

A   **B**

Figure 3-33. A. Choledochal cyst with a short, fusiform dilatation. B. Extensive choledochal cyst involving the entire extrahepatic biliary tree and bifurcation.

extrahepatic biliary tree and the bifurcation (Figure 3-33B). Type III choledochal cysts or choledochoceles are choledochal cysts that protrude into the lumen of the duodenum. Choledochal cysts and especially choledochoceles are frequently associated with anomalous pancreaticobiliary ductal union. As a result, drainage of the bile duct may be sluggish due to a sump phenomenon, which predisposes to sludge and stone formation. Similarly, pancreatic ductal drainage may be impaired, predisposing to attacks of pancreatitis. Although the traditional management of choledochal cysts is surgical resection, endoscopic sphincterotomy and deroofing of the cyst provide immediate drainage in cases of biliary sepsis or acute pancreatitis. Because choledochal cysts are associated with an increased risk of bile duct malignancy, consideration should be given to surgical resection, even when endoscopic therapy has relieved the acute problem.

Biliary cysts are reported much more frequently in Asian populations than in the West. The female to male ratio is 3–4 to 1. Most cases are diagnosed in childhood or young adulthood. Figure 3-34 shows the Todani classification of biliary cysts. A prominent feature of choledochal cysts is anomalous pancreaticobiliary ductal union. This occurs in 40% or more of cases (some report 100%). There also appears to be an association between anomalous ductal union and the incidence of biliary malignancies. The presentation of choledochal cysts in infants is often indistinguishable from biliary atresia (jaundice, hepatomegaly). In adults, presentations range from an incidental finding during cholecystectomy or abdominal imaging to biliary obstruction (cholangitis, jaundice) and recurrent pancreatitis. Untreated, biliary obstruction and sepsis can result in liver abscess, biliary cirrhosis, and portal hypertension. There is a strong association between choledochal cysts and the development of

Figure 3-34. The Todani classification of biliary cysts. A. Type IA, localized extrahepatic. Type IB, segmental dilation. Type IC, diffuse or cylindrical dilation. B. Type II, extrahepatic diverticulum. Type III, choledochocele. C. Type IVA, multiple intrahepatic and extrahepatic cysts. Type IVB, multiple extrahepatic cysts only. D. Type V, solitary intrahepatic cyst.

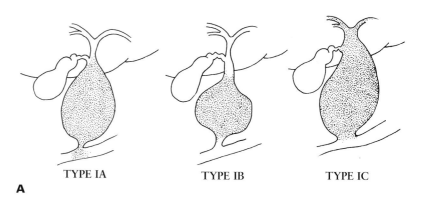

TYPE IA   TYPE IB   TYPE IC

A

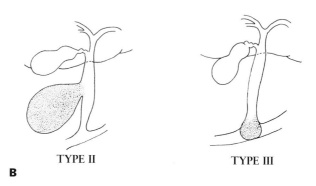

TYPE II   TYPE III

B

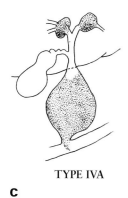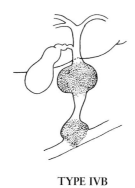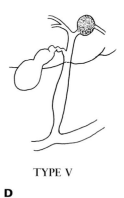

TYPE IVA   TYPE IVB   TYPE V

C   **D**

malignancy, usually adenocarcinoma. Surgical resection of the chole-dochal cyst reduces this risk of malignancy but does not completely eliminate it because the entire pancreaticobiliary tree appears to be pre-disposed to undergo malignant transformation.

Hemobilia

Hemorrhage into the biliary tree produces blood clots that have a typical appearance on cholangiography (Figure 3-35). Although the bile ducts may become filled with clot, it is rare for hemobilia to cause mechanical biliary obstruction. Leung and his colleagues in Hong Kong have used the throm-bolytic agent, urokinase, to dissolve obstructing blood clot in a patient with hemobilia. Hemobilia is one of the causes of obscure GI bleeding. It may be suspected if there is a likely cause (Table 3-3), or if blood or blood clot is seen exiting the duodenal papilla. There is little an endoscopist can do other than demonstrating the abnormality. Persistent hemobilia is an indication for celiac arteriography to pinpoint the bleeding vessel. In select-ed cases, embolization of bleeding vessels, tumors, and aneurysms can stop the bleeding. Occasionally, surgery is needed to investigate and treat per-sistent hemobilia.

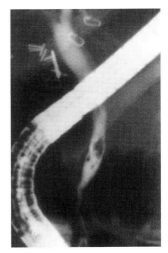

Figure 3-35. Hemobilia. Filling defects on the cholangiogram are caused by blood clot.

Pancreas Divisum

In pancreas divisum, failure of fusion of the dorsal and ventral segments of the embryonic pancreas results in two separate ductal systems (Figure 3-36). The ventral duct, entered through the main duodenal papilla, is small and sometimes absent. The majority of the exocrine pancreas

Table 3-3. Causes of hemobilia

Surgery
Penetrating trauma*
Instrumentation*
    Liver biopsy
    Percutaneous transhepatic cholangiography (guidewire trauma)
    Endoscopic retrograde cholangiopancreatography (guidewire trauma)
Blunt trauma*
Hepatoma
Bile duct tumor
Choledocholithiasis (rare)

*Usually associated with pseudoaneurysm formation.

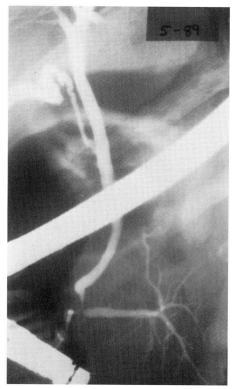

A

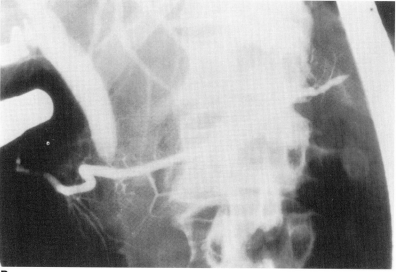

Figure 3-36. A. Ventral duct system in pancreas divisum. B. Dorsal duct system in pancreas divisum.

B

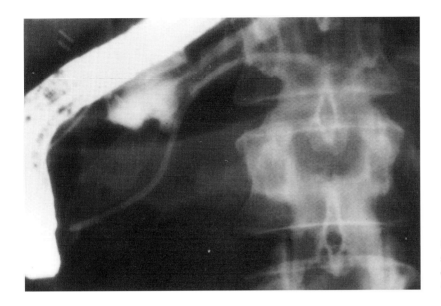

Figure 3-37. Endoscopic stenting of the dorsal pancreatic duct in pancreas divisum.

secretions drain through the dorsal duct, which exits into the duodenum through the minor duodenal papilla. In the United States and Europe, pancreas divisum occurs in 7–8% of the population. Pancreas divisum occurs in considerably fewer individuals of Asian and African origin, possibly in the range of 2–3%. Of interest, divisum anatomy occurs in up to 25% of cases of annular pancreas, another congenital anomaly in which the pancreas may partially encircle the descending duodenum. Pancreatitis and small tumors may occasionally interrupt the normal communication between the dorsal and ventral pancreatic ducts, creating an *acquired divisum* state.

The vast majority of patients with pancreas divisum have a gland that functions normally, but some patients with pancreas divisum have chronic abdominal pain or chronic, relapsing pancreatitis. The relationship between pancreas divisum anatomy and pancreatitis is hotly debated, but a hypertensive dorsal duct secondary to minor papilla stenosis or dysfunction—or a dominant stricture—can undoubtedly cause pancreatic pain and pancreatitis. Lans demonstrated that dorsal duct stenting (Figure 3-37) of patients with pancreas divisum and recurrent pancreatitis reduced the frequency of episodes of pancreatitis and the need for hospitalization. Lehman reported that minor papilla sphincterotomy provided relief in about 80% of divisum patients with recurrent pancreatitis. On the other hand, patients who had pain syndromes without objective signs of pancreatitis or those with advanced chronic pancreatitis had a much lower response rate. In limited studies, endoscopic stenting for pancreatic-type pain in patients with pancreas divisum but otherwise normal-looking ducts had distinctly mixed results. Only half derived symptomatic benefit,

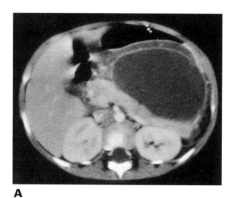

A

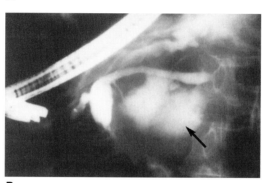

B

Figure 3-38. A. Computerized tomogram of abdomen, showing a pancreatic pseudocyst, which appears as the large, fluid-filled, thick-walled cavity occupying much of the right side of the image. B. Pancreatic pseudocyst (arrow) demonstrated to be in communication with the main pancreatic duct (ERCP).

and often this was short-lived. This procedure cannot be recommended for routine use. It has been suggested by several ERCP experts that endopancreatic therapy should be used only in the setting of clinical trials until better data are available.

Pancreatic Pseudocyst

Pancreatitis may be complicated by the formation of walled-off, fluid-filled, cystic cavities (Figure 3-38A). The majority are in communication with the pancreatic ductal system. Continuous exocrine secretion ensures that these cysts remain full as long as they remain in communication with the pancreatic duct (Figure 3-38B). Pseudocysts may occur at any site from the head to the tail of the pancreas and vary enormously in size. The contents also vary from pure fluid to thick, necrotic debris. The walls of pseudocysts may be very thin or thicker than a centimeter. The latter often have large blood vessels coursing through the walls, which has significance for the endoscopist who is considering endoscopic pseudocyst decompression.

ERCP has a useful role to play in defining the anatomy of pseudocysts and planning appropriate management. An algorithm for the management of pseudocysts developed at Duke University Medical Center uses the pancreatogram to predict whether or not percutaneous drainage alone will be likely to resolve the pseudocyst. Simply stated, pseudocysts are unlikely to resolve spontaneously when there is continued communication with the main pancreatic duct, especially if the duct has been disrupted downstream from the communication. On the other hand, pseudocysts not in communication with the main pancreatic duct are likely to resolve with aspiration or temporary catheter drainage, or both.

Several endoscopic techniques have been used to facilitate decompression of pancreatic pseudocysts. Pancreatic stents may be employed to decompress high-pressure ducts in the presence of papillary stenosis or spasm, dominant ductal strictures, or disruptions. Alternatively, a nasopancreatic drain may be placed, which provides the additional benefit of continuous aspiration. In both cases, the hope is that lowering the pressure in the ductal system will allow communication to cease spontaneously or will empty a pseudocyst if it can be reached directly. Finally, in highly selected cases, pancreatic pseudocysts can be decompressed directly into the lumen of the stomach (cyst gastrostomy) (Figure 3-39) or duodenum (cyst duodenostomy). *This procedure should be performed only by experienced endoscopists with appropriate surgical backup.* The most suitable pseudocysts for decompression by endoscopically created fistulae are thin-walled structures of water density that clearly impinge on the wall of the stomach or duodenum. Because thick-walled pseudocysts are often vascular, their puncture is associated with an increased risk of bleeding, which may be torrential and life-threatening.

To reduce the risk of inadvertently puncturing a large blood vessel in the process of opening up the pseudocyst with a cautery device (e.g., needle knife), several useful techniques have been developed. Where the technology is available, endoscopic ultrasound can clearly define the anatomy of the pseudocyst and its wall (Figure 3-40). When duodenoscopes with built-in ultrasound transducers become routinely available, targeted incision of pseudocysts through safe sites should become routine. For the present, however, the endoscopic ultrasound scope has to be withdrawn and another scope (usually a duodenoscope) introduced to perform the decompression procedure. Howell has recently described a useful technique that requires cheaper and more readily available technology. A 22 Fr needle is advanced through a plastic sleeve into the pseudocyst (Figure 3-41). First, fluid withdrawn for cytology and microbiology is inspected to ensure that blood is not present. Fresh blood in the aspirate suggests that a vessel has been punctured and that this is an unsuitable area for further manipulation. If the aspirate is not bloody, the needle can be withdrawn and a needle knife incision performed at the same site. Once the orifice has been created by electrocautery, the plastic catheter is advanced into the cavity to maintain access. Using a guidewire passed through the catheter, pigtail stents are placed to maintain drainage. Some authors recommend that a

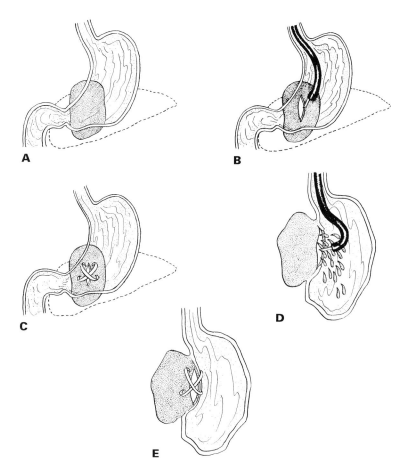

Figure 3-39. Endoscopic cyst gastrostomy. A. Coronal section showing relationship of stomach, pancreas (dotted line), and pseudocyst (gray structure). B. Using a needle knife catheter, a small slit is created to produce a communication between the pseudocyst and the posterior wall of the stomach. C. The opening is kept open and draining by inserting two pigtail plastic stents (the curly lines). D. Pseudocyst puncture (releasing fluid) seen in sagittal section. E. Stent placement between stomach and pseudocyst (sagittal section).

nasocystic drain should also be placed to allow lavage of the cavity and subsequent contrast imaging to be performed.

It is important that the decision to perform endoscopic pseudocyst drainage be made after full consultation with colleagues in surgery and radiology because the endoscopic approach carries the potential for limiting subsequent radiologic access for percutaneous drainage if the pseudocyst reaccumulates or fails to drain. Also, if there is major ductal disruption downstream from the pseudocyst, it is unlikely that transmural endoscopic drainage will be any more successful than percutaneous aspiration or catheter drainage. The pigtail stents placed in the pseudocyst should be removed after several weeks to limit the risk of stent migration. Stents that migrate into the pseudocyst cavity are inaccessible to the endoscopist and can only be removed by surgery. If the patient is asymptomatic, migrated stents are usually left in place. Evidence of sepsis or persistent pain related to foreign body reaction is an indication for surgery

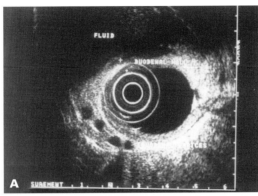

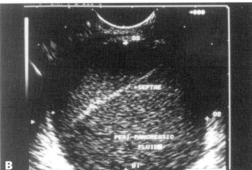

Figure 3-40. Endoscopic ultrasound defines the anatomy of the pancreatic pseudocyst and its wall. A. Endoscopic ultrasound in descending duodenum showing pseudocyst (fluid) and nearby varices (to be avoided during puncture). B. Endoscopic ultrasound demonstrating fluid-filled pseudocyst plus septum, suggesting that the fluid is loculated. (Courtesy of Dr. R. Hawes.)

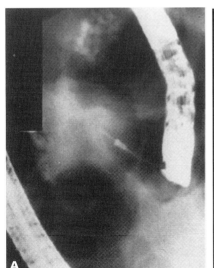

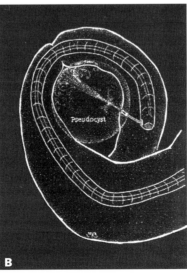

Figure 3-41. A. A radiograph shows a Howell needle used to puncture pancreatic pseudocysts. The needle is seen emerging laterally from the tip of the duodenoscope and puncturing the pseudocyst (opacified with radiographic contrast medium). B. A schematic of the radiograph. (Reprinted with permission from DA Howell, RF Holbrook, JJ Bosco, et al. Endoscopic needle localization of pancreatic pseudocysts before transmural drainage. Gastrointest Endosc 1993;39:693.)

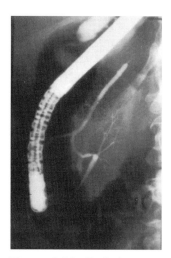

Figure 3-42. Typical pancreatic ductal disruption caused by trauma.

to retrieve the stents and deal with the residual pseudocyst. It should be remembered that cystic tumors occasionally masquerade as pancreatic pseudocysts. It is a wise precaution to send fluid aspirated from pseudocysts for cytologic examination. Fluid from mucinous cystic tumors may contain large concentrations of carcinoembryonic antigen. Assay for carcinoembryonic antigen should be considered if this diagnosis is being entertained. Pseudocysts containing multiple septae or loculi should be considered suspicious for underlying neoplasia; for example, microcystic adenomas are often misdiagnosed as pseudocysts.

Pancreatic Duct Strictures

Strictures of the pancreatic duct may be solitary or multiple, benign or malignant. One of the most important missions for the endoscopist performing ERCP is to pursue possible pancreatic malignancy aggressively.

Sometimes, there is little doubt about the etiology of a pancreatic ductal stricture. Following blunt or penetrating trauma, the duct may be partially or totally obstructed by a tight stricture (Figure 3-42). In chronic pancreatitis of any etiology, multiple strictures (*chain of lakes*) are almost certain to be benign in origin (Figure 3-43). Often, the most worrisome strictures are solitary. Adult patients without a clear reason for pancreatitis (e.g., gallstones, alcohol, trauma) who present with pancreatic pain or relapsing pancreatitis and a solitary stricture should be considered to have malignancy until proved otherwise.

A variety of endoscopic methods are available to obtain tissue from pancreatic duct strictures, including brush cytology (performed over a guidewire) and aspiration biopsy, usually employing a sclerotherapy-type needle. If the pancreatic duct is sufficiently dilated, standard biopsy forceps can be advanced into the duct to obtain tissue. Malignant cells may also be recovered from pure pancreatic juice recovered after secretin stimulation. A variety of molecular biology techniques are currently being evaluated for sensitivity and specificity in diagnosing malignancy from such samples. If a mass can be seen at the site of the stricture on ultrasound or CT scanning, an attempt may be made to obtain tissue by percutaneous biopsy under

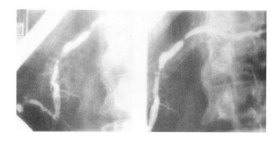

Figure 3-43. Typical strictures of chronic pancreatitis (chain of lakes appearance).

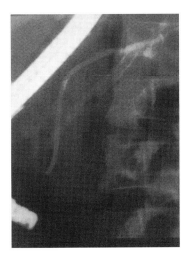

Figure 3-44. Endoscopic stenting of benign pancreatic duct strictures.

radiologic guidance. Published studies suggest that even the best results from pure juice studies, brush cytology, direct biopsy, and percutaneous needle biopsy aspiration yield only 50–75% positive results in malignancy. What might be considered the definitive diagnostic test, however, direct handling of the pancreas by a surgeon and directed biopsy, has a sensitivity not much better than 80%.

When significant suspicion of a malignant stricture exists despite negative investigations, sometimes it is justifiable to resect the majority of the pancreas, as in the Whipple procedure, in the hope of completely removing an early cancer. Because the prognosis of primary adenocarcinoma of the pancreas is extremely poor (1-year survival is approximately 5% in many published series), it is essential to make the diagnosis as early as possible. It is hoped that evolving techniques for studying pancreatic juice, cytologic specimens, and tissue biopsies will render speculative surgery redundant.

Endoscopic stenting of the pancreatic duct for benign strictures (Figure 3-44) has been reported by numerous authors to provide good symptomatic relief for periods ranging from months to years. Lehman has recently pointed out that these trials often suffer from poor data. In particular, the length of follow-up is extremely variable, clinical improvement may be poorly characterized, and most reports ignore the clinical course following stent removal. Of interest, one European expert has been using expandable metal mesh stents for persistent benign pancreatic duct strictures. There are limited data on the efficacy of this approach. Accordingly, expandable metal mesh stents for benign pancreatic strictures cannot be recommended for routine use at present.

Stenting for pancreatic duct strictures is not without complications, which include migration into the pancreatic duct and pancreatic edema and fibrosis due to local irritation and obstruction of side branches (Figure 3-45). The frequency of pancreatic stent–induced ductal irregularity and

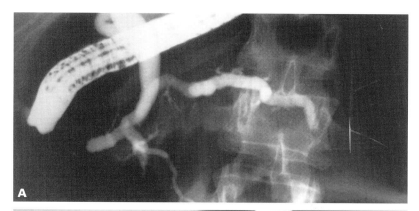

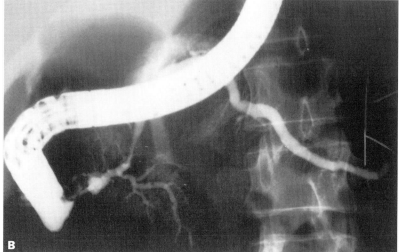

Figure 3-45. A. Pancreatic duct strictures before stenting. B. Severe changes in the side branches of the duct in the head of the pancreas following only 1 week's stenting.

narrowing is as high as 80% in patients who start out with an otherwise normal duct. In an 8-month study, Lehman has shown that one-third of these changes fail to resolve fully. These findings have been duplicated in a dog model. Pancreatic stenting for benign strictures should be considered a short-term repair in younger patients, most of whom eventually require a surgical drainage procedure for long-term relief of symptoms. Symptomatic patients with pancreatic duct strictures of the head and body of the gland associated with upstream ductal dilatation are best managed by side-to-side pancreaticojejunostomy (Puestow procedure). This leaves the strictured area (and its associated side branch abnormalities) in place to cause continued pain, however. If the stricture is sufficiently left of the midline, resection of the stricture with the tail of the pancreas may be preferable. Strictures without significant ductal dilatation upstream have a less predictable response to all types of surgical and nonsurgical therapy.

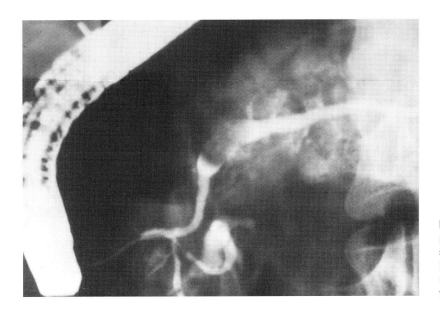

Figure 3-46. Obstructing pancreatic duct stone. Pressure of a contrast injection has caused tissue disruption (acinarization) "upstream" from the obstruction.

Pancreatic Duct Stones

Stones in the pancreatic duct may be the cause of chronic pancreatitis or simply an epiphenomenon reflecting the underlying pathologic process, but they also can obstruct exocrine outflow (Figure 3-46). It is easy to believe that this results in chronic pain or continuing pancreatitis. Because some patients improve clinically when their pancreatic stones are removed surgically, an association seems likely.

Endoscopic removal of pancreatic duct stones is technically difficult. It usually requires pancreatic sphincterotomy followed by stone extraction using balloons or baskets. When this direct approach fails, a stent or nasopancreatic drain can be placed and ESWL administered. There is enormous variation in the reported technical success of pancreatic stone clearance in the published literature (27–100%). In patients in whom stone clearance was complete, however, the majority (perhaps 85%) had symptomatic improvement for a mean follow-up of up to 2 years. Manipulation of stones in the pancreatic duct carries a risk of causing pancreatitis (one-third of patients undergoing ESWL in one study developed infection). When pancreatic stone extraction is impossible or incomplete, placing a stent across the pancreatic duct sphincter may prevent obstruction of exocrine outflow. Because pancreatic stent placement may be associated with unpleasant complications, including infection, stent migration, pseudocyst formation, occlusion, and ductal abnormalities, long-term stenting is to be avoided. It is definitely a short-term maneuver that may be helpful in predicting the outcome of more definitive drainage. Not all stones in the pancreas arise from the pancreatic duct. Occasionally, a gall-stone migrates into the pancreatic duct instead of exiting through the papil-la, particularly if there is a long, shared common channel at the ampulla. This phenomenon may cause gallstone pancreatitis.

Ampullary Tumors

Tumors of the ampulla of Vater constitute only 5% of the pancreaticobil-iary pathology encountered by endoscopists, but they have certain unique features that merit review. Histologically, ampullary growths range from benign adenomas to frank carcinomas. There are also largely benign growths that comprise neuroendocrine elements (e.g., carcinoid, ganglio-neuroma). The progression from benign to malignant can be difficult to determine. Some histologically benign tumors behave in a rather malignant fashion, with local recurrence after endoscopic or surgical excision. The sampling error inherent in endoscopic biopsy means that one can never be sure that ampullary mass with dysplasia does not contain frank carcinoma. For this reason, the treatment of ampullary masses is often determined as much by their behavior as by their histology.

Locally recurrent tumors are thought to have malignant potential and are therefore an indication for pancreatic resection (e.g., with the Whipple procedure). Multiple villous tumors may be found in the duodenum in familial polyposis syndromes, such as Gardner's syndrome. The duodenal papilla is sometimes the site of a tumor. Because the tumors are too numer-ous to resect endoscopically or surgically, frequent endoscopic surveillance with biopsy is appropriate to look for dysplasia, indicating a trend toward malignant transformation. Ampullary tumors are usually exophytic and quite soft. If they are sufficiently friable, recurrent minor bleeding may result in iron deficiency anemia, which brings the disorder to light. Ampullary tumors may not obstruct biliary flow until the mass has become quite large. Obstructive jaundice is therefore a late feature. Abnormal LFTs (especially alkaline phosphatase) and biliary dilatation on ultrasound may be stimuli to investigation while the tumor is still small. The *silver stool* sign, said to be pathognomonic of ampullary tumors, is a rarity.

The usual landmarks for cannulating the bile duct and pancreatic duct are frequently absent in the presence of an ampullary tumor, but the open-ing to the bile duct is often near the apex of the tumor (Figure 3-47). Gen-tle probing with an ERCP cannula or soft (hydrophilic) guidewire frequently yields access. In my experience, the pancreatic duct is harder to find; cannulation is largely a matter of trial and error. This is not a major problem, however, because pancreatography is rarely required to make the diagnosis or perform endoscopic treatment.

What treatments are available for ampullary tumors? Palliation of obstructive jaundice can be achieved by placing a stent if biliary cannulation

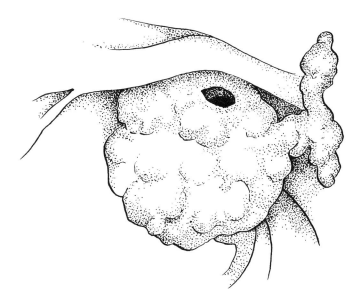

Figure 3-47. When an ampullary tumor is present, access to the bile duct is often near the tumor's apex.

is successful. When the endoscopic approach fails, another option is a combined procedure using a radiologically placed guidewire. Once the endoscopist retrieves the tip of the guidewire from the duodenum and brings it back up through the endoscope channel, it can be used to facilitate catheter and stent placement in the normal fashion. As always in malignant obstruction of the bile duct, the largest available endoprosthesis (stent) should be placed (normally, 10 Fr or 11.5 Fr). Endoscopic sphincterotomy—or in this case, more correctly, endoscopic papillotomy—can be used to open up the distal end of the bile duct. This technique has fallen from favor, though, because the relief of obstruction is often short lived (due to regrowth of the tumor) and there is a significant risk of hemorrhage when cutting through tumor. There is also the concern that sphincterotomy in this setting may allow a potentially resectable tumor to metastasize so that it becomes unresectable. Certainly, a surgical opinion should first be obtained if there is any prospect that the patient will be offered local or radical surgical resection.

A group in Hamburg, Germany published their experience of endoscopic snare papillectomy in 1993. In this technique, the papilla is encircled using a standard endoscopic snare (Figure 3-48). The papillary mass is then removed using electrocautery. This is a technique for experts only. The German authors had good results but, as expected, there were a number of local recurrences of the tumor and some complications, including pancreatitis. Clearly, one benefit of this aggressive approach is that a large piece of tissue is obtained for histologic analysis. Even if the tumor appears to be grossly and macroscopically benign, frequent screening endoscopies should be planned to ensure that the

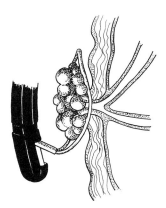

Figure 3-48. Schematic of an endoscopic snare papillectomy.

Figure 3-49. Separate openings to the bile duct and pancreatic duct after snare papillectomy. When the duodenal wall heals after snare papillectomy, two separate orifices to the bile duct and pancreatic duct (p) are clearly seen. (Reprinted with permission from KF Binmoëller, S Bonaventura, K Ramsperger, N Soehendra. Endoscopic snare excision of benign adenomas of the papilla of vater. Gastrointest Endosc 1993;39:127.)

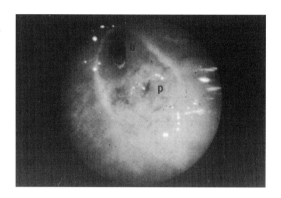

tumor does not recur locally. There are no hard and fast guidelines regarding screening, but evaluations of the papilla using a side-viewing endoscope at 6 and 12 months followed by annual examinations thereafter would be appropriate. Electrocautery in the vicinity of the papilla always creates the risk of stenosis of one or both of the ductal orifices (Figure 3-49). Temporary stenting of both orifices after the procedure appears to reduce the risk. A similar problem can arise after laser photocoagulation of papillary lesions, a technique reported to be beneficial in expert hands.

Occasionally, papillary tumors grow into the pancreatic or bile duct without obvious mass effect externally. These small, often pedunculated tumors may cause intermittent biliary obstruction or relapsing pancreatitis from transient obstruction of the ampulla or relevant duct. The presence of such a tumor may be suggested by a mobile filling defect at ERCP in either duct (Figure 3-50). Sometimes endoscopic sphincterotomy is necessary to open up the ampulla to gain access for biopsy or cytology brushing. When small, mobile masses "pop out" after sphincterotomy, endoscopic snare excision may be possible. These ductal growths tend to recur locally.

Most papillary tumors are seen in middle-aged and elderly patients. Often, pancreatic resection for cure is impossible, so palliation becomes the major therapeutic issue. Patients with papillary tumors often have an extended survival (several years or more) with repeated endoscopic stenting. The stent can generally be left in place until there is clinical or biochemical evidence of occlusion, requiring extraction and replacement. The natural history of ampullary malignancies is to grow progressively. Published studies suggest that in 10–20% of patients with ampullary cancer, the tumor will eventually obstruct the duodenum, necessitating decompressive surgery. In patients who are fit for surgery, a double bypass procedure is indicated, namely gastroenterostomy and choledochoenterostomy. With the advent of laparoscopic surgery, it has been possible to bypass the duodenal obstruc-

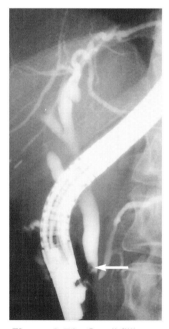

Figure 3-50. Small filling defect in the distal common bile duct due to an intra-ampullary tumor.

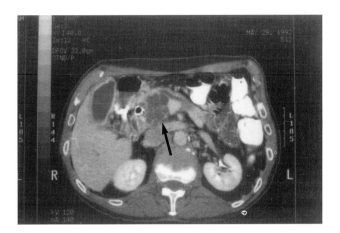

Figure 3-51. Computed tomographic scan showing microcystic adenoma of the head of the pancreas.

tion by laparoscopic gastroenterostomy. If the patient has an intact gall-bladder, cholecystenterostomy may also be performed laparoscopically to decompress the biliary tree. Continued endoscopic stenting is impractical in patients with an enlarging duodenal mass because the area becomes progressively more difficult to access for stent exchange.

Unusual Pancreatic Tumors

The most common primary malignancy involving in the pancreas is adenocarcinoma, but the ERCP endoscopist should be aware of a variety of unusual malignancies that may occur in the pancreas. Cystic neoplasms often masquerade as pancreatic pseudocysts. Microcystic adenomas tend to be multiloculated (Figure 3-51) and are associated with relapsing pancreatitis. Cystic tumors may be serous or mucinous. Mucinous cystic neoplasms of the pancreas have only recently been recognized as a discrete entity. These mucin-producing tumors, which often arise in the uncinate process of the pancreas, may present with relapsing pancreatitis. On CT scan, the pancreatic duct is grossly dilated, and at ERCP, mucinous material may be seen extruding from the pancreatic duct orifice, which is unusually prominent. With the exception of gross mucin-secreting tumors, ERCP is not especially useful in confirming a diagnosis of cystic neoplasm, but it is of help in defining the pancreatic ductal anatomy for surgical resection.

The pancreas may be the seat of primary lymphoma and a variety of connective tissue tumors. Tumors metastatic to the pancreas are unusual but should be considered when the pancreas appears to be the seat of a "second primary." A primary lymphoma should be considered when there is a large pancreatic mass on CT with peripancreatic lymphadenopathy.

Traditionally, it has been considered important to distinguish lymphoma from carcinoma because the former is likely to respond to chemotherapy or radiotherapy and is often associated with longer survival. Of interest, the last two patients I have seen with primary pancreatic lymphoma survived 5 and 6 months, an outlook no better than adenocarcinoma of pancreas. Spectacular remissions do occur, however, and therefore aggressive pursuit of this diagnosis remains appropriate.

One of the greatest diagnostic challenges of the pancreas is to detect tumors arising from the islets of Langerhans. Islet cell tumors usually come to light because of symptoms related to endocrine activity (e.g., insulinoma, gastrinoma, VIPoma, glucagonoma). These tumors may be very small indeed, resisting all efforts to localize them radiologically. ERCP is almost never helpful in this search. Modern CT technique can identify certain lesions as small as 5 mm in the pancreas. Endoscopic ultrasound, which can inspect the pancreatic head through the duodenum and the body and tail through the gastric antrum, is said to be even more sensitive. If an islet cell tumor can be accurately located, the surgeon's job is much easier. With intraoperative ultrasound probes, the area of interest can be minutely inspected and the appropriate resection performed. A recent innovation with considerable promise is intraductal ultrasound of the pancreas using very small ultrasound probes. At present, the tissue penetration of intraductal ultrasound is extremely limited, but technological advances are bound to improve this rapidly. Similarly, magnetic resonance imaging using gated techniques to compensate for respiratory motion is now yielding valuable information about pancreatic ductal anatomy and certain parenchymal lesions.

Hemosuccus Pancreaticus

Hemosuccus pancreaticus is the exotic term used to describe the pancreatic equivalent of hemobilia. Blood exiting the pancreatic duct orifice is most commonly associated with a splenic artery aneurysm that is in communication with the pancreatic duct in the tail of the gland. An abdominal CT scan may show a cystic structure near the spleen, which may be calcified (Figure 3-52). Arteriography is usually needed to define the lesion and embolize it. In cases of failed embolization, surgery will be required.

Guidewires

Modern diagnostic and therapeutic ERCP have benefited greatly from the development of a variety of guidewires (Figure 3-53). The standard 0.035-inch diameter wire, the core of the standard stenting system, lacks the

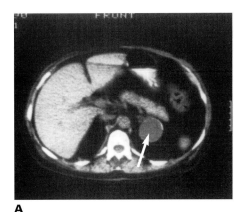

A

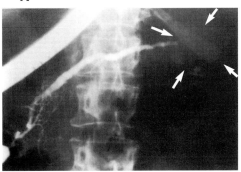

B

Figure 3-52. A. Computerized tomogram of abdomen, showing a pseudoaneurysm of the splenic artery. B. Plain abdominal radiographic image of a pseudoaneurysm of the splenic artery (the faintly calcified cystic structure in the tail of the pancreas).

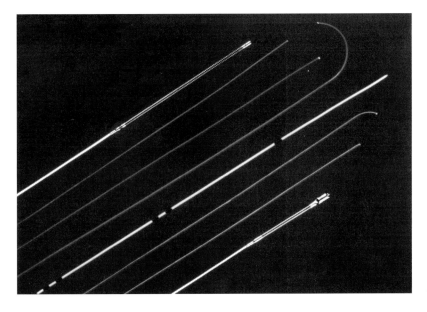

Figure 3-53. A variety of endoscopic guidewires.

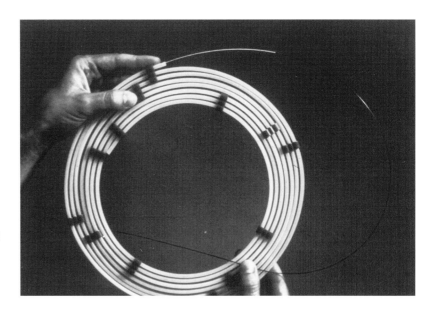

Figure 3-54. Teflon-coated guidewire. The major advance in guidewire technology has probably been polymer coating.

smoothness and flexibility to negotiate irregular strictures or tight bends. The smallest wire in routine use is the 0.018-inch wire, which is used to introduce biliary manometry catheters into the bile duct. These wires are floppy and easily dislodged. The 0.021- and 0.025-inch wires are stiff enough to be useful in negotiating tight strictures and pass through most endoscopic accessories used in ERCP that admit a guidewire.

Probably the major advance in guidewire technology has been polymer coating (Figure 3-54). The usual polymer is Teflon, which can be applied as a painted surface or as a uniform coat. Teflon-coated wires provide electrical insulation, an important consideration when using wire-guided catheters to perform sphincterotomy. At least one accessory company has produced a coated guidewire that is guaranteed to provide electrical insulation during sphincterotomy. This is useful when it is imperative to maintain access to the bile duct following sphincterotomy, as is often the case following difficult cannulation. Many coated guidewires are hydrophilic; that is, they absorb water, making their surface slippery. The flexibility of coated wires, combined with their slippery surface, make them ideal for negotiating strictures and odd angles. To enhance the visibility of these wires, the manufacturers have added refinements, such as radiopaque tips (made of platinum or similar dense metal). Another useful modification has been partial coating of the wires. Completely coated guidewires, once rendered slippery by saline priming, are harder to handle than normal (uncoated) wires and are difficult to hold on to using the elevator of the duodenoscope. Coating only the distal tip (the business

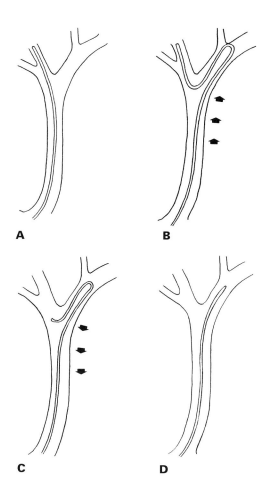

Figure 3-55. Using the guidewire to "knuckle" into the desired duct. A. Wire preferentially enters the right intrahepatic duct system. B. Additional wire is advanced into bile duct knuckles into left main hepatic duct. C. As the wire is withdrawn slowly, it tends to snake out of the left main hepatic duct. D. If the maneuver is performed carefully, the tip of the wire remains in the left main hepatic duct at the end of the procedure.

end) of the wire leaves the majority of the wire less slippery and more easily handled.

The flexibility of modern guidewires can be used to advantage in cannulating the desired duct or ducts in the liver. If, for example, the guidewire repeatedly enters the right intrahepatic system, pushing in an additional length can cause the body of the wire to knuckle into the desired duct (Figure 3-55). When the wire is withdrawn, the tip may be left in the desired system. The torque-stable biliary guidewire is as close to being the Holy Grail of ERCP as anything. Although torque-stable guidewires work well on the laboratory bench, they tend to lose their magic when deployed through an endoscopic channel. This is undoubtedly due to the loss of mechanical advantage that is inevitable when using endoscopic accessories in the bile duct. Because guidewires cannot be sterilized effectively between procedures, they should be discarded and not reused.

Needle Knife Papillotomy

Needle knife papillotomy (NKP) is a method for gaining access to the bile duct by incising overlying tissues. It is often used as an alternative to standard endoscopic sphincterotomy when deep cannulation of the bile duct fails.

The needle knife is a plastic catheter with a bare wire at the tip. The wire is used to apply cautery directly to the surface mucosa and underlying tissues. Because the current density at the tip of the wire is very high (being inversely proportional to the area of contact) the needle knife is a powerful and potentially dangerous tool. NKP should only be performed by endoscopists with considerable experience of endoscopic sphincterotomy. I share the consensus view that NKP should be reserved solely for therapeutic access in cases requiring biliary decompression, such as cholangitis, gallstone pancreatitis, and some ampullary and pancreatic head tumors. It should not be used as an alternative to skill at biliary cannulation. The technique I prefer is to use a needle knife with a very thin wire, applying current as a series of brush strokes, usually in a downward (caudad) direction.

The two safest situations in which to use NKP are (1) release of an impacted stone in gallstone pancreatitis and (2) cutting down onto a stent for sphincterotomy in the B-II patient. When a stone is impacted at the ampulla, it is often impossible to advance the tip of a sphincterotome or guidewire beyond it to gain deep access to the common bile duct. The papilla is usually bulging, with the stone visible in the orifice. The appearance is often likened to the head of a baby crowning during labor (Figure 3-56). A cut down onto the stone in the 12 o'clock position using the needle knife usually frees the impacted stone, which pops out into the duodenum. This is often followed by a gratifying gush of bile or pus. The opening can then be cannulated for extension of the cut using standard endoscopic sphincterotomy technique. If the papillary fold is deroofed using a needle knife, the bile duct may not be immediately apparent. A little pool of bile may be the only clue to its whereabouts. The opening created by NKP may be gently probed using a flexible (soft-tip) coated guidewire in the hope of finding the bile duct. Firmer, uncoated wires may cause local trauma or perforation. In one-third to one-half of cases of NKP used blindly (i.e., not over a stent or down onto a stone), a second procedure may be needed to obtain bile duct access. Biliary drainage should not be delayed in patients with cholangitis. Percutaneous cholangiography and drain or stent placement should be performed without delay in failed NKP cases if sepsis is the major indication for biliary access. A needle knife papillotome should be

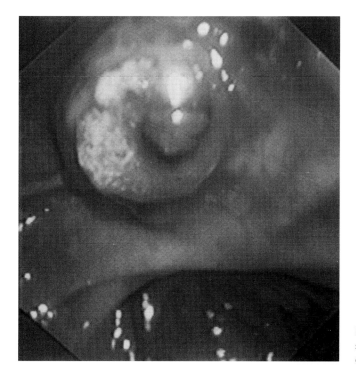

Figure 3-56. Impacted stone emerging from the duodenal papilla.

available in every busy endoscopy unit, but NKP must be used selectively by skilled endoscopists only.

Stents and Stenting

Since the introduction of 10 Fr biliary stenting in 1980, stent technology has become universally available and applied (Figures 3-57 and 3-58). There is a large and ever increasing list of indications for endoscopic stenting both in the biliary tree and pancreas. When plastic stents were introduced for endoscopic use, few would have thought that there was much room for innovation in design, but more stent designs are available now than ever before, probably a reflection of the lack of an ideal plastic stent.

A common indication for endoscopic stenting is mechanical obstructive jaundice. Carr-Locke (personal communication) found the following distribution of causes of jaundice in a personal series of more than 1,000 patients: gallstones (36%), pancreatic cancer (22%), intrahepatic cholestasis (14%), bile duct cancer (8%), ampullary tumors (7%), metastases

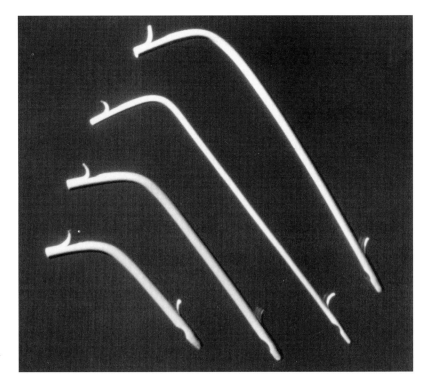

Figure 3-57. A variety of polyethylene biliary stents of Amsterdam design (i.e., flaps and side holes top and bottom). (Courtesy of Wilson-Cook Medical, Inc., Winston-Salem, NC.)

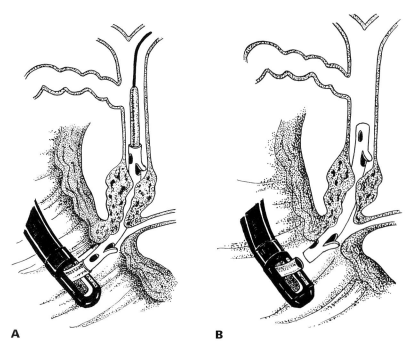

Figure 3-58. A. Placement of a polyethylene biliary stent across a low bile duct stricture using the guidewire, inner catheter, and stent with pusher tube technique. The guidewire and inner catheter provide the required stiffness for stent insertion. B. Once the stent is appropriately positioned across the stricture, the inner catheter and wire are removed, leaving the stent in place to provide biliary drainage.

A   **B**

compressing the bile duct (4%), benign biliary stricture in chronic pancreatitis (2%), dilated bile duct (only) (2%), traumatic common bile duct stricture (2%), sclerosing cholangitis (2%) and unknown (1%). The
distribution of the 41% of patients with malignancy was pancreatic (22%),
biliary (8%), ampullary (7%), and metastases to the portal nodes (4%).
More than 80% were unresectable on imaging. Since the introduction of
large-caliber (10 Fr and greater) biliary stents by the Amsterdam group,
plastic endoprosthesis placement has become the mainstay of palliative
therapeutic endoscopy in malignant jaundice. Unfortunately, little progress
has been made in dealing with the problem of stent occlusion. The use of
antibiotics or antibiotic- and bacteriostatic-impregnated stents has not pre-
vented the clogging phenomenon. The use of gallstone dissolution agents,
mucolytic agents, and choleretic agents has been similarly unimpressive.

One solution to the problem of plastic stent occlusion has been the introduction of metallic expandable mesh stents. The United States medical
community has the most experience with the Schneider Wallstent (Schneider [USA], Inc., Minneapolis, MN), which is delivered on an 8 Fr system;
it expands to 30 Fr in fully expanded form, with a final length of 68 mm
(Figure 3-59). Some potential technical difficulties are associated with
deploying the Wallstent, mainly due to shortening of the stent as it
expands. Care must be taken not to leave the distal end of the stent close
to the papilla, where it may fail to open and cause biliary obstruction. Similarly, deployment of the proximal end is restricted in a small intrahepatic
biliary duct. Initial studies in Europe revealed the problems of late
ingrowth with tumor (Figure 3-60) and mucosal hypertrophy (10%). The
Wallstent Study Group in the United States has conducted a randomized
trial of the Wallstent versus conventional 10 Fr biliary stents for palliating
malignant obstructive jaundice. Of 182 patients randomized, 94 got Wallstents and 88 got plastic stents, with a high success rate of positioning
(97% and 95%, respectively). Half the cancers were pancreatic, with less-
er numbers of biliary, metastatic, and other tumors. Three percent of plastic stents occluded within 30 days; no Wallstents occluded. Late stent
complications after 30 days were sludge occlusion in 25% of plastic stents
(5% in Wallstents) but tumor ingrowth or overgrowth in 10% of the Wallstent group only, making for overall complication rates of 16% for Wallstents and 31% for plastic stents ($P < 0.05$). Life-table analysis showed no
difference in survival, but the mean time to stent occlusion was prolonged
to 132 days for Wallstents; plastic stents were almost three times more likely to block than Wallstents. A study in Holland showed similar results in
terms of a lower complication rate and prolonged patency, as well as significant impact on cost effectiveness.

Other expandable metal stents, such as Palmaz, Strecker (not available
in the United States), Gianturco Z stent (Wilson-Cook Medical, Inc., Winston-Salem, NC) (Figure 3-61), and nitinol coil (e.g., EndoCoil, CR Bard,
Billerica, MA), are slowly being approved for endoscopic use in the biliary
tree. When uncoated metal stents occlude with tumor, we usually deal
with this by inserting a plastic stent across the obstruction. A more expen-

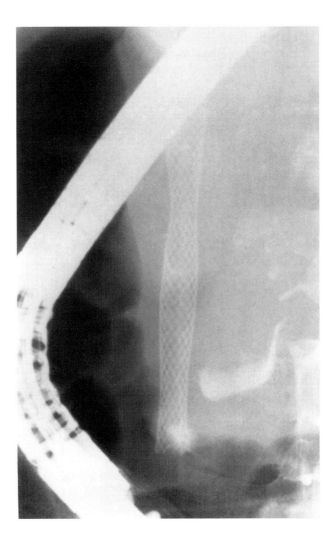

Figure 3-59. Wallstent fully deployed across bile duct stricture.

sive alternative is to place a second metal stent inside the first one. The difficult problem of tumor ingrowth may have an ingenious solution in the form of photodynamic therapy, but expandable metal mesh stents with plastic coatings may prevent the problem altogether. Preliminary experience of coating metal stents for use in the esophagus in malignant dysphagia has been promising.

There has been a natural reluctance to place expandable metal mesh stents in benign biliary strictures because of their permanence. Until the long-term results of clinical trials are available, this use of metal stents must be considered experimental.

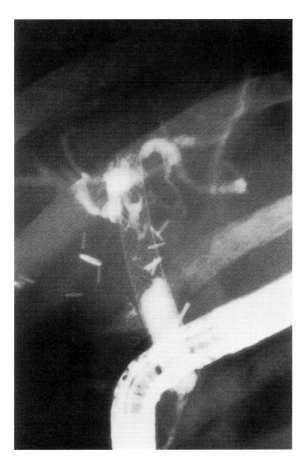

Figure 3-60. Tumor ingrowth occluding expandable metal mesh stent.

Stents in the Pancreatic Duct

It has become clear that biliary stents are unsuitable for routine use in the pancreas, where stent migration is a major problem. To address the problem of stent migration, stents have been designed with large external pigtails and multiple flaps to resist migration into the pancreatic duct. When a long pancreatic stent is required (e.g., for a stricture in the body or toward the tail of the pancreas), an appropriately shaped stent, to fit the ductal anatomy, is preferable. Pancreatic duct stents can cause significant ductal and side branch abnormalities (see Figures 3-45A and B). Because these abnormalities generally occur in the vicinity of the stent (rather than upstream), it is likely that they are due to local irritation and mechanical obstruction of the side branches. Fortunately, the majority of these changes are partially or totally reversible. Pancreatic stents should be considered a short-term remedy for dominant strictures or hypertonic sphincters, but they are unsuitable for longer-term management.

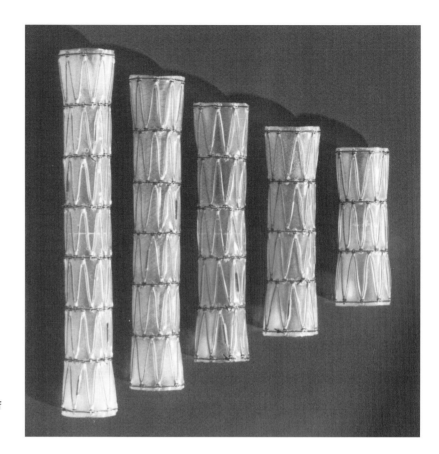

Figure 3-61. Coated Gianturco Z stents. Initially used for esophageal stenoses, this design is being modified for use in the biliary tree. (Courtesy of Wilson-Cook Medical, Inc., Winston-Salem, NC.)

Tissue Diagnosis of Malignant Strictures

The appropriate management of strictures in the biliary tree and pancreas depends on accurate tissue diagnosis. This can be maddeningly difficult. The gold standard, open biopsy of a suspicious mass or stricture at laparotomy, has at best a sensitivity of around 80%. Considerable attention has focused on techniques for obtaining cytology and histology at ERCP. Ryan and Bardorf compared flow cytometry for DNA content with brush cytology for detecting malignancy in pancreatic and biliary strictures. They found that the addition of flow cytometry to routine cytology increased the diagnostic yield. In addition, patients with a diploid cell population survived significantly longer (mean, 8.9 months) than those with predominantly aneuploid cells (mean, 3.0 months). Ferrari et al. found that standard brush cytology had a specificity and positive predictive value of 100% but a sensitivity of only 56.2%. In an effort to increase the yield, Mohandas et al. dilated biliary strictures to 10 Fr, which they found to have the desired effect. In an elegant study, Baron et al. compared the cellular yield when the brush was removed from its sheath with the yield when it was left in place. Withdrawing the brush through the sheath markedly reduced the yield of cells. This loss could be compensated for by salvage cytology, when the catheter was flushed to remove adherent cells.

Biopsy specimens offer a large quantity of tissue for analysis. Lo et al. have compared their diagnostic yield with forceps, brush cytology, and bile aspiration in 49 malignant and 25 benign strictures. The sensitivity for forceps biopsy in biliary strictures was 71% overall, being lower in pancreatic (58%) than nonpancreatic (84%) tumors. Inexplicably, they had a miserably poor yield of cytology from brushing (14%) and bile (8%). Kubota et al. used malleable forceps in 43 patients, only 14 of whom had a prior sphincterotomy. Adequate samples were obtained in 41 of 43 patients. Positive histologic diagnosis was made in 16 of 18 cholangiocarcinomas (89%) and 10 of 14 (71%) pancreatic carcinomas. There were no false-positive results.

A genetic alteration at codon 12 in the *c-K-ras* gene has been found in the majority of pancreatic carcinomas. In a retrospective analysis of paraffin-embedded tissue specimens obtained by percutaneous fine needle aspiration, DNA from 47 patients was amplified by polymerase chain reaction. Mutant *c-K-ras* oncogene was positive in 20 of 36 (56%) pancreatic cancer patients. Overall, the mutation was positive in 18 of 25 cases with malignant cytology, 2 of 8 with atypical cytology, and 0 of 3 with benign cytology. A recently published study from Brussels reported detecting the *c-K-ras* mutation in 83% of 24 patients with pancreatic carcinomas, with no false-positive results (Van Laethem et al.). Endoscopic ultrasound-guided fine needle aspiration biopsy is likely to enhance our ability to target suspicious lesions in the pancreas, distal common bile duct, and adjacent lymph nodes and to obtain tissue for marker studies.

Sphincter of Oddi Manometry

Sphincter of Oddi manometry is used to determine whether or not SOD contributes to postcholecystectomy pain syndrome, relapsing pancreatitis, or obscure abdominal pain of indeterminate origin when other investigations have drawn a blank. Sphincter of Oddi manometry is performed using a 200-cm long polyethylene catheter with an outer diameter of 1.7 mm and a luminal diameter of 0.5 mm (Figure 3-62). Recording apertures are spaced at 2-mm intervals, starting 5 mm from the tip. The catheter, which is perfused with water at a flow rate of 0.25 ml per minute, is advanced through the instrument channel of the duodenoscope. Because it is technically difficult to freely cannulate the bile duct with this soft and easily bent catheter alone, we like to advance it over a thin (0.018-inch) guidewire positioned in the bile duct during prior cannulation with a standard ERCP catheter.

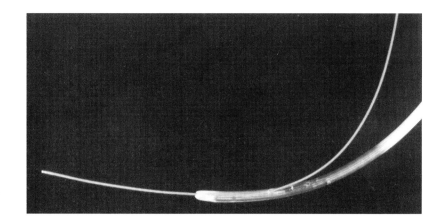

Figure 3-62. Biliary manometry catheter as used to measure sphincter of Oddi pressures.

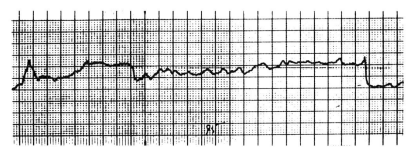

Figure 3-63. Biliary manometry pressure tracing showing sustained elevation of sphincter of Oddi pressure. Time is shown on the X-axis and pressure measurement on the Y-axis.

After recording baseline common bile duct pressure for 1–2 minutes, the catheter is slowly withdrawn in 2- to 3-mm increments, exposing each of the recording apertures (ports) to the sphincter segment. Recordings are performed at each station for at least 1 minute. To test reproducibility, these pull throughs are repeated two or three times. The mean basal sphincter pressure is averaged from the maximal basal pressure reading at each station during at least two pull throughs. Basal sphincter pressures greater than 40 mm Hg above intraduodenal pressure are considered abnormal (Figure 3-63). Operators should be aware of phasic contractions that are superimposed on the basal sphincter tone: they occur about four times each minute and last 4–5 seconds. Phasic wave contractions measure 150 ± 60 mm Hg in amplitude. These phasic waves are normally directed in an antegrade direction. Retrograde propagation is seen in some patients with suspected SOD. Intravenous administration of CCK-octapeptide decreases basal pressure in the sphincter of Oddi and abolishes phasic wave contractions in normal individuals. In some patients with SOD, CCK-octapeptide causes a paradoxical increase in basal sphincter of Oddi pressure. Increased phasic wave activity (*tachyoddia*) has been shown to occur after intravenous morphine injection. This may explain attacks of pain and abnormal LFT results seen in some patients after morphine administration.

Suggested Reading

Papillary Stenosis and Sphincter of Oddi Dysfunction

Botoman VA, Kozarek RA, Nowell LA, et al. Long term outcome after ES in patients with biliary colic and suspected sphincter of Oddi dysfunction. Gastrointest Endosc 1994;40:165.

Geenen JE, Hogan WJ, Dodds WJ, et al. The efficacy of endoscopic sphincterotomy after cholecystectomy in patients with sphincter of Oddi dysfunction. N Engl J Med 1989;320:82.

Hawes RH, Tarnasky PR. Endoscopic manometry of the sphincter of Oddi: its usefulness for the diagnosis and treatment of benign papillary stenosis. Gastrointest Endosc 1996;43:536.

Hogan WJ, Geenen JE. Biliary dyskinesia. Endoscopy 1988;20:179.

Kozarek RA. Biliary dyskinesia: are we getting any closer to defining a clinical entity? Gastrointest Endosc Clin North Am 1993;3:167.

Common Bile Duct Stone Removal

MacMathuna P, White P, Clarke E, et al. Endoscopic sphincteroplasty: a novel and safe alternative to papillotomy in the management of bile duct stones. Gut 1994;35:127.

May SR, Cotton PB, Edmunds SEJ, Chang W. Removal of stones from the bile duct at ERCP without sphincterotomy. Gastrointest Endosc 1993;39:749.

Onken JE, Brazer SR, Eisen GM, et al. Predicting the presence of choledocholithiasis in patients with symptomatic cholelithiasis. Am J Gastroenterol 1996; 91:762.

Mechanical Lithotripsy

Chung SCS, Leung JWC, Leung HT, Li AKC. Mechanical lithotripsy of large common bile duct stones. Br J Surg 1991;78:1448.

Shaw MJ, Mackie RD, Moore JP, et al. Results of a multicenter trial using a mechanical lithotripter for the treatment of large bile duct stones. Am J Gastroenterol 1993;88:730.

Contact Lithotripsy

Ell C, Hochberger J, May A, et al. Laser lithotripsy of difficult bile duct stones by means of a rhodamine-6G laser and an integrated automatic stone-detection system. Gastrointest Endosc 1993;39:755.

Jakobs R, Maier M, Kohler B, Reimann JF. Peroral laser lithotripsy of different intrahepatic and extrahepatic bile duct stones: laser effectiveness using an automatic stone-tissue discrimination system. Am J Gastroenterol 1996; 91:468.

Neuhaus H, Hoffman W, Gottlieb K, Classen M. Endoscopic lithotripsy of bile duct stones using a new laser with automatic stone recognition. Gastrointest Endosc 1994;40:708.

Prat F, Fritsch J, Chaury AD, et al. Laser lithotripsy of difficult biliary stones. Gastrointest Endosc 1994;40:290.

Mirizzi Syndrome

Binmoeller KF, Thonke F, Soehendra N. Endoscopic treatment of Mirizzi syndrome. Gastrointest Endosc 1993;39:532.

Binnie NR, Nixon SJ, Palmer KR. Mirizzi syndrome managed by endoscopic stenting and laparoscopic cholecystectomy. Br J Surg 1992;79:647.

Stents for Bile Duct Stones

Bergman JJGHM, Rauws EAJ, Tijssen JGP, et al. Biliary endoprostheses in elderly patients with endoscopically irretrievable CBD stones: report on 117 patients. Gastrointest Endosc 1995;42:195.

Johnson SK, Geenen JE, Venu RP, et al. Treatment of non-extractable common bile duct stones with combination ursodeoxycholic acid plus endoprostheses. Gastrointest Endosc 1993;39:528.

Surgery for Bile Duct Stones

Davidson BR, Lauri A, Horton R, et al. Outcome of surgery for failed endoscopic extraction of common bile duct stones in elderly patients. Annu Rev R Coll Surg Engl 1994;76:320.

Bile Duct Leaks

Kozarek RA, Ball TJ, Patterson DJ, et al. Endoscopic treatment of biliary injury in the era of laparoscopic cholecystectomy. Gastrointest Endosc 1994;40:10.

Biliary Strictures

Kozarek RA. Endoscopic approach to biliary strictures. Gastrointest Endosc Clin North Am 1993;3:261.

Pugliese V, Conio M, Nicolo G, et al. Endoscopic retrograde forceps biopsy and brush cytology of biliary strictures: a prospective study. Gastrointest Endosc 1995;42:520.

Sclerosing Cholangitis

Broome U, Olsson R, Loof L, et al. Natural history and prognostic factors in 305 Swedish patients with primary sclerosing cholangitis. Gut 1996;38:610.

Cappell MS. Hepatobiliary manifestations of the acquired immune deficiency syndrome. Am J Gastroenterol 1991;86:1.

Chen LY, Goldberg HI. Sclerosing cholangitis: broad spectrum of radiographic features. Gastrointest Radiol 1984;9:39.

Craig DA, MacCarthy RL, Wiesner RH, et al. Primary sclerosing cholangitis: value of cholangiography in determining prognosis. AJR 1991;157:959.

Daly CA, Padley SP. Sonographic prediction of a normal or abnormal ERCP in suspected AIDS-related sclerosing cholangitis. Clin Radiol 1996;51:618.

Jansen PL, Sanders JB. Primary sclerosing cholangitis: an unresolved enigma. Scand J Gastroenterol 1992;194(Suppl):76.

Wiesner RH, Grambsch PM, Rhodes JM, et al. Primary sclerosing cholangitis: natural history, prognostic factors and survival analysis. Hepatology 1989; 10:430.

Endoscopic Retrograde Cholangiopancreatography in Relation to Laparoscopic Cholecystectomy

Chan ACW, Chung SCS, Wyman A, et al. Selective use of preoperative ERCP in laparoscopic cholecystectomy. Gastrointest Endosc 1996;43:212.

Davids PHP, Rauws EAJ, Coene PPLO, et al. Endoscopic stenting for post-operative biliary strictures. Gastrointest Endosc 1992;38:12.

Kozarek RA, Ball TJ, Patterson DJ, et al. Endoscopic treatment of biliary injury in the era of laparoscopic cholecystectomy. Gastrointest Endosc 1994; 40:10.

Kozarek RA, Gannan R, Baerg R, et al. Bile leak after laparoscopic cholecystectomy. Arch Intern Med 1992;152:1040.

Manoukian AV, Schmalz MJ, Geenen JE, et al. Endoscopic treatment of problems encountered after cholecystectomy. Gastrointest Endosc 1993;39:9.

Santucci L, Natalini G, Sarpi L, et al. Selective endoscopic retrograde cholangiography and preoperative bile duct stone removal in patients scheduled for laparoscopic cholecystectomy: a prospective study. Am J Gastroenterol 1996;91:1326.

Choledochal Cysts

Chaudhary A, Dhar P, Sachdev A, et al. Choledochal cysts—differences in children and adults. Br J Surg 1996;83:183.

Samuel M, Spitz L. Choledochal cyst: varied clinical presentations and long-term results of surgery. Eur J Pediatr Surg 1996;6:78.

Todani T, Wanatabe Y, Narusue M, et al. Congenital bile duct cysts. Classification, operative procedures and review of 37 cases including cancer arising from choledochal cyst. Am J Surg 1977;134:263.

Zimmon DS, Falkenstein DB, Manno BV, et al. Choledochocele: radiologic diagnosis and endoscopic management. Gastrointest Radiol 1978;3:349.

Hemobilia

Curet P, Baumer R, Roche A, et al. Hepatic hemobilia of traumatic or iatrogenic origin: recent advances in diagnosis and therapy, review of the literature from 1976 to 1981. World J Surg 1984;8:2.

Floyd WN, Jr. Radiologic aspects of hemobilia. South Med J 1981;74:829.

Sanblom P, Saegesser F, Mirkovitch V. Hepatic hemobilia: hemorrhage from the intrahepatic biliary tract: a review. World J Surg 1984;8:41.

Pancreas Divisum

Kozarek RA, Ball TJ, Patterson DJ, et al. Endoscopic approach to pancreas divisum. Dig Dis Sci 1995;40:1974.

Lans JI, Geenen JE, Johanson JF, et al. Endoscopic therapy in patients with pancreas divisum and acute pancreatitis: a prospective, randomized, controlled clinical trial. Gastrointest Endosc 1992;38:430.

Lehman GA, Sherman S. Pancreas divisum: diagnosis, clinical significance and management alternatives. Gastrointest Endosc Clin North Am 1995;5:145.

Pancreatic Pseudocyst

Ahearne PM, Baillie J, Cotton PB, et al. An endoscopic retrograde cholangiopancreatography (ERCP)-based algorithm for the management of pancreatic pseudocysts. Am J Surg 1992;163:111.

Cremer M, Deviere J, Engelholm L. Endoscopic management of cysts and pseudocysts in chronic pancreatitis: longterm follow-up after 7 years of experience. Gastrointest Endosc 1989;35:1.

Howell DA, Holbrook RF, Bosco JJ, et al. Endoscopic needle localization of pancreatic pseudocysts before transmural drainage. Gastrointest Endosc 1993;39:693.

Lawson JM, Baillie J. Endoscopic therapy for pancreatic pseudocysts. Gastrointest Endosc Clin North Am 1995;5:181.

Pancreatic Duct Strictures

Howell DA, Beveridge RP, Bosco J, et al. Endoscopic needle aspiration biopsy at ERCP in the diagnosis of biliary strictures. Gastrointest Endosc 1992; 38:531.

Jowell PS. Assessment of pancreatic duct strictures. Gastrointest Endosc Clin North Am 1995;5:125.

Pancreatic Duct Stones

Alhalel R, Haber GB. Endoscopic therapy of pancreatic stones. Gastrointest Endosc Clin North Am 1995;5:195.

Kozarek RA, Ball TJ, Patterson DJ, et al. Endoscopic pancreatic duct sphincterotomy: indications, techniques and analysis of results. Gastrointest Endosc 1994;40:592.

Guidewires

Baillie J. The Hydrophilic Guidewire. In J Barkin, CA O'Phelan (eds), Advanced Endoscopy (2nd ed). New York: Raven, 1994;277.

Jacob L, Geenen JE. ERCP guidewires (a review). Gastrointest Endosc 1996;43:57.

Needle Knife Papillotomy

Foutch PG. A prospective assessment of results for needle-knife papillotomy and standard endoscopic sphincterotomy. Gastrointest Endosc 1995;41:25.

Biliary and Pancreatic Stenting

Davids PHP, Groen AK, Rauws EAJ, et al. Randomized trial of self-expanding metal stents vs polyethylene stents for distal malignant biliary obstruction. Lancet 1992;340:1488.

Dertinger S, Ell C, Fleig WE, et al. Long-term results using self-expanding metal stents for malignant biliary obstruction. Gastroenterology 1992;102:A310.

Deviere J, Bueso H, Baize M, et al. Complete disruption of the main pancreatic duct: endoscopic management. Gastrointest Endosc 1995;42:445.

Huibregtse K, Katon RM, Coene PP, Tytgat GNJ. Endoscopic palliative treatment in pancreatic cancer. Gastrointest Endosc 1986;32:334.

Ponchon T, Bory RM, Hedelius F, et al. Endoscopic stenting for pain relief in chronic pancreatitis: results of a standardized protocol. Gastrointest Endosc 1995;42:452.

Raijman I, Lalar E, Marcon NE. Photodynamic therapy for tumor ingrowth through an expandable esophageal stent. Gastrointest Endosc 1995;41:73.

Seitz U, Vadeyar H, Soehendra N. Prolonged patency with a new-design Teflon biliary prosthesis. Endoscopy 1994;26:478.

Sung JJY, Chung SCS, Tsui C-P, et al. Omitting side holes in biliary stents does not improve drainage of the obstructed biliary system: a prospective, randomized trial. Gastrointest Endosc 1994;40:321.

Tissue Diagnosis of Malignant Strictures

Baron TH, Lee JG, Wax TD, et al. An in vitro, randomized, prospective study to maximize cellular yield during bile duct brush cytology. Gastrointest Endosc 1994;40:146.

Ferrari AP Jr, Lichtenstein DR, Slivka A, et al. Brush cytology during ERCP for the diagnosis of biliary and pancreatic malignancies. Gastrointest Endosc 1994;40:140.

Kubota Y, Takaoka M, Tani K, et al. Endoscopic transpapillary biopsy for diagnosis of patients with pancreaticobiliary ductal strictures. Am J Gastroenterol 1993;88:1700.

Lo SK, Venegas R, Chen J, Doo E. A prospective, blinded evaluation of five cytologic sampling methods for diagnosing neoplastic biliary strictures [abstract]. Gastrointest Endosc 1995;41:404A.

McGuire DE, Venu RP, Brown RD, et al. Brush cytology for pancreatic carcinoma: an analysis of factors influencing results. Gastrointest Endosc 1996;44:300.

Mohandas KM, Swaroop VS, Gullar SU, et al. Diagnosis of malignant obstructive jaundice by bile cytology: results improved by dilating the bile duct strictures. Gastrointest Endosc 1994;40:150.

Ryan ME, Bardorf MC. Comparison of flow cytometry for DNA content and brush cytology for detection of malignancy in pancreaticobiliary strictures. Gastrointest Endosc 1994;40:133.

Van Laethem J-L, Vertangen P, Deviere J, et al. Detection of c-K-ras gene codon 12 mutations from pancreatic duct brushings in the diagnosis of pancreatic tumors. Gut 1995;36:781.

Vilmann P, Hancke S, Henriksen FW, Jacobsen GK. Endoscopic ultrasound–guided final needle aspiration biopsy of lesions in the upper gastrointestinal tract. Gastrointest Endosc 1995;41:230.

4

Evolving Techniques

One of the last frontiers of GI endoscopy is the small intestine. It has been fortunate for endoscopists that only 2% of pathology affecting the entire GI tract involves the small bowel from the ligament of Treitz to the ileocecal valve. Routine small bowel radiology has a low yield of positive findings in patients with obscure GI bleeding (about 5%; enteroclysis increases this to around 10%). Radioisotope bleeding scans, Meckel's diverticulum scan, and angiography also have a role to play. Increasingly, endoscopy includes the small intestine. Standard esophagogastroduodenoscopy (EGD) can reach the second or third part of the duodenum. It is possible to survey the entire duodenum and a small distance into the proximal jejunum using a pediatric colonoscope passed by mouth. At colonoscopy, a skilled practitioner can consistently intubate the ileocecal valve and inspect the distal 10–20 cm of ileum in perhaps 80% of cases. The remainder of the small intestine, however, has remained inaccessible to endoscopists until recently. Endoscope design has improved significantly over the last 20 years, so it is now possible to build endoscopes that permit inspection of the small intestine.

Push Enteroscopy

Two types of enteroscope are available: the push and sonde instruments. Push enteroscopes are significantly longer than a standard gastroscope, with lengths ranging from 200–250 cm. The original push enteroscope designs were based on fiberoptic technology, but charged couple device chip scopes are now available. Push enteroscopy is significantly different from standard EGD because of the tendency of the long scope to loop in the stomach (Figure 4-1). For this reason, most examinations are performed with an overtube to straighten the instrument in the stomach. With skilled use of the overtube, the small bowel can be examined up to 120 cm beyond the ligament of Treitz.

Patients do not enjoy swallowing overtubes; they are bulky and cause an unpleasant sensation of a foreign body in the upper esophageal sphincter. As a result, many patients need deeper sedation for enteroscopy than for

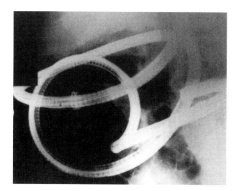

Figure 4-1. Fluoroscopic picture of a push enteroscope in position in the small bowel.

standard EGD. It is more comfortable, and safer, to advance the overtube over a well-lubricated 44 Fr Maloney dilator. The enteroscope is passed like a standard gastroscope and the tip negotiated through the stomach and pylorus into the proximal duodenum. It is usually possible to advance the scope into the second or third part of the duodenum before significant looping occurs. In anticipation of this, the straightening overtube can be advanced into position in the stomach as soon as the pylorus has been intubated. It should be remembered that overtubes are associated with risk of trauma to the hypopharynx, upper esophageal sphincter, and the esophagus itself, so considerable care should be taken not to apply major force against resistance.

It is not always necessary to use an overtube; in my own experience, it is possible to achieve a satisfactory examination without an overtube in about one-half of cases. When small bowel motility makes it difficult to perform enteroscopy, a pharmacologic agent may be administered to inhibit this, such as glucagon, atropine, or one of its derivatives. The twists and turns of the proximal small intestine are not predictable; the endoscopist must be prepared to use a combination of inputs to cautiously negotiate whatever he or she encounters. The aim is to keep the tip of the endoscope oriented in the middle of the lumen. Because it is virtually impossible to avoid superficial trauma caused by direct contact with the tip or pressure from slide-by maneuvers, it is vital to perform the inspection as the endoscope advances rather than during withdrawal.

The mucosa of the duodenum and jejunum tends to be sticky, especially after a prolonged fast. This renders the process of insufflation (to open up the lumen) rather tedious. I have found that injecting sterile water with simethicone (antifoaming agent) through the instrument channel of the scope periodically helps loosen the folds and renders them easier to separate by insufflation.

Patients who have had prior abdominal surgery causing adhesions or who have other pathology rendering the bowel less compliant than usual present a particular technical challenge. If major resistance to advancing the scope is encountered, and it is not clearly due to looping in the stomach, consideration should be given to abandoning the procedure because the risk of trauma, including perforation, is significant. Where available, it is a wise precaution to perform enteroscopy under fluoroscopic surveillance. This allows the endoscopist to check for looping, to ascertain the likely position of the endoscope tip, and to ensure that the overtube is used correctly.

Published studies suggest that up to a third of examinations for obscure GI bleeding yield a significant abnormality on enteroscopy. These include vascular malformations (telangiectasia), which comprise 80% of lesions identified, diverticula, and benign and malignant tumors. The newer push enteroscopes have instrument channels large enough to admit biopsy forceps, polypectomy snares, and other instruments. Using them, it is possible to apply effective endoscopic therapy for telangiectasia. If a suspect diverticulum or tumor is identified, however, it is likely that the case will proceed to laparotomy to resect the lesion.

It is important to be able to mark the site of the lesion for subsequent identification, which can be extremely difficult in the case of the small bowel. The standard methods for identifying sites of lesions (e.g., local injection of India ink, placement of endoscopic clips) may not be available or may be rendered impossible by the length or position of the endoscope. As an alternative, the endoscopist may elect to repeat enteroscopy in the operating room at the time of surgery (intraoperative endoscopy). When the endoscopist identifies the lesion, he or she can transilluminate the bowel wall at that point to provide a target area for the surgeon.

Intraoperative endoscopy is a useful technique that is practiced infrequently due to the difficulty endoscopists encounter when working in the operating room. Operating room rules may specify that a sterile endoscope be used. Standard GI endoscopes are rarely sterilized (e.g., by ethylene oxide), because it is an expensive and time-consuming procedure. Because the GI tract is hardly a sterile environment, it makes little sense to require absolute sterility (unless the scope is being inserted through an enterotomy incision). The presence of an endotracheal tube with an inflated cuff in the upper airway may render it technically difficult to pass a large-bore overtube. An overtube is unnecessary, however, because the surgeon can reduce loops in the stomach manually and help to feed the endoscope through the bowel. It should be remembered that push enteroscopy carries some risk of trauma, including perforation and postprocedure ileus.

Sonde Enteroscopy

An older method of small bowel enteroscopy is to weight a thin endoscope and allow it to pass through the small bowel largely by peristalsis (Figures 4-2A and B). This technique is called sonde enteroscopy. Sonde scopes are usually advanced through a nostril rather than the mouth. The patient is

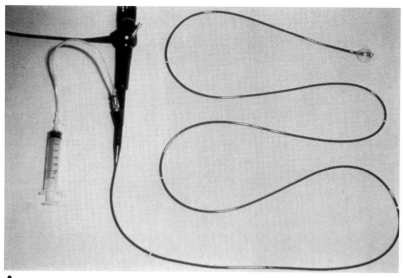

A

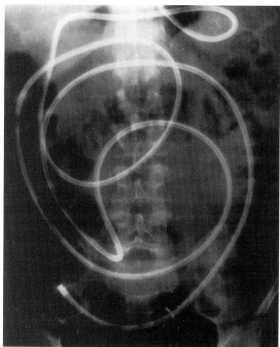

B

Figure 4-2. A. Sonde enteroscope laid out on a table. B. Fluoroscopic view of sonde enteroscope passed down to the ileum. (Courtesy of Dr. Blair Lewis.)

asked to swallow the scope when it is in the hypopharynx and in this way it advances into the stomach, much like a nasogastric tube. Although sonde scopes can be allowed to advance beyond the stomach solely by motility, a preferred method is to help it on its way by passing a gastroscope alongside it and using forceps to pull or drag the tip of the endoscope into the duodenum. Once the tip of the sonde scope is positioned in the proximal duodenum, a balloon on the distal end is inflated to encourage peristalsis, which carries the instrument through the small bowel. Normal peristaltic action allows the scope to advance slowly but at a steady rate. If the enteroscope is being advanced solely by peristalsis from the stomach, the patient is first positioned in the right lateral position. It is customary to administer a prokinetic agent, such as metoclopramide or cisapride, to enhance peristaltic action. Once the endoscope has reached the descending duodenum (either by a natural means or with endoscopic help), the patient is encouraged to lie on his or her left side. This position increases the chances that it will pass quickly through the duodenum into the upper jejunum.

Sonde enteroscopy is a time-consuming procedure; it is not unusual to spend 6 hours or more waiting for the tip of the scope to reach the distal ileum. Sometimes the sonde scope fails to get this far. The procedure should be performed in a comfortable room with sufficient distractions, such as television or magazines, to make the patient's waiting tolerable. The patient should undergo fluoroscopy from time to time to ascertain the likely position of the tube tip. The time taken for the tube to pass through the entire small intestine is quite variable. Repeated administration of a prokinetic agent may be required to encourage motility. The patient may complain of abdominal cramping pain, for which analgesia is rarely required, or nausea and vomiting, which may respond to an antiemetic agent.

Once fluoroscopy confirms that the tip of the sonde endoscope is in the desired position in the ileum, the endoscopist is ready to perform enteroscopy. The balloon on the tip is deflated and the instrument slowly pulled back. There is no tip deflection available on these instruments, so the view is distinctly limited, but the combination of slow withdrawal and repeated inflation and deflation of the balloon allows much of the small intestine to be inspected. Should an abnormality be identified, the approximate position should be confirmed on fluoroscopy.

Sonde scopes have the limitation of having no facility for biopsy or the passage of other accessories, such as brushes and injection needles. The combination of Sonde and push enteroscopy, however, allows inspection of the entire small bowel, significantly increasing the endoscopist's contribution to the investigation of obscure GI bleeding and abnormal small bowel radiology. Lewis compared the yield of push and sonde enteroscopy in 504 patients: push enteroscopy alone yielded diagnosis in 19% of patients; Sonde enteroscopy increased this by a further 28%. Of 191 patients with small bowel angiodysplasia, 47% had lesions within the reach of the pediatric colonoscope. Of 16 small bowel tumors, 68% were diagnosed at push enteroscopy and 32% by sonde technique. The volume of patients who might benefit from enteroscopy is generally too small in the average practice to justify the purchase of dedicated endoscopes. Accordingly, the majority of enteroscopies will continue to be performed at tertiary referral centers.

Endoscopic Ultrasound

What Is Endoscopic Ultrasound?

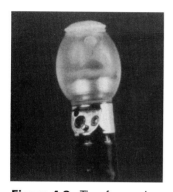

Figure 4-3. Tip of an endoscopic ultrasound scope showing the transducer housed in a water balloon. (Courtesy of Olympus Corp., Lake Success, NY.)

One of the most exciting recent developments in GI endoscopy is endoluminal ultrasound imaging, usually referred to as endoscopic ultrasound (EUS). The concept is simple: an ultrasound transducer is engineered into the tip of a flexible endoscope (Figure 4-3) to allow imaging of the wall of the gut and its adjacent structures. Technically, this presents an enormous challenge. Several types of ultrasound transducers can be used, most commonly the radial and linear array designs. Tissue penetration (i.e., the depth of imaging and resolution) depends on the frequency of the ultrasound used. The standard EUS frequencies are 7, 12.5, and 25 MHz. In general, as frequency increases so does the resolution but at the expense of depth of penetration. One of the many fascinating aspects of EUS is its ability to delineate the layers of the bowel wall as well as adjacent structures (Figure 4-4), including blood vessels and lymph nodes (Figures 4-5 and 4-6). In addition to these structures, it can provide unique views of the heart through the esophagus and the biliary tree and pancreas through the stomach and duodenum (Figure 4-7). EUS has literally added a new dimension to gut imaging.

EUS has proved to be a more useful diagnostic tool in the upper GI tract than in the colon (with the exception of the rectum). This technique allows visualization of the layers of the wall of the esophagus, stomach, and duodenum and adjacent structures. The technology readily identifies varices

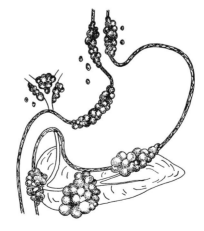

Figure 4-4. The spectrum of lesions in the upper gastrointestinal tract amenable to imaging by endoscopic ultrasound. These include esophageal, gastric, and duodenal masses (both intrinsic and extrinsic), their related lymph nodes, and ampullary, pancreatic, and biliary tumors.

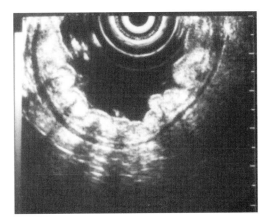

Figure 4-5. Endoscopic ultrasound delineates layers of the bowel wall as well as adjacent structures.

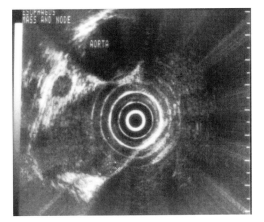

Figure 4-6. Endoscopic ultrasound scan from the lumen of the esophagus showing a mass involving the esophageal wall with adjacent lymphadenopathy. The proximity of the aorta to the esophagus and this lesion are clearly demonstrated.

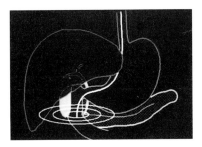

Figure 4-7. Schematic of endoscopic ultrasound of head of pancreas.

masquerading as thickened gastric folds (Figure 4-8) and helps to determine the nature of submucosal lesions. Benign lesions (e.g., lipomas, leiomyomas) are seen to be encapsulated, with the layers of the bowel wall remaining intact. Malignant tumors can be seen to breach these layers. EUS is particu-

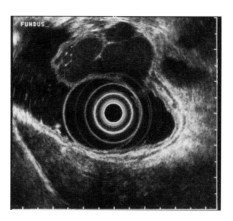

Figure 4-8. Endoscopic ultrasound is an excellent way to identify varices masquerading as large folds in the gastric fundus. (Reprinted with permission from G Caletti, A Ferrari. Endoscopic unltrasound. Endoscopy 1996;28:156.)

larly useful in staging esophageal and gastric cancers. Not only is the extent of wall invasion detectable, but enlargement and altered consistency of local lymph nodes may indicate local metastasis. EUS also has increased the utility of the tumor node metastasis (TNM) classification of GI malignancies. The extrahepatic biliary tree can be examined through the wall of the duodenal bulb and proximal descending duodenum, and this is one way to identify common bile duct stones prior to endoscopic retrograde cholangiopancreatography. The gastric antrum and medial wall of descending duodenum offer a variety of unique EUS views of the pancreas and peripancreatic lymph nodes. Blood vessels can also be seen, which is useful in the assessment of tumor resectability. A variant of EUS is the use of small ultrasound probes that can be passed through the instrument channel of conventional endoscopes. These have been used successfully to define tumors and localize optimum sites for endoscopic pseudocyst drainage.

Targeted Biopsies Using Endoscopic Ultrasound

One of the exciting prospects of evolving EUS technology is targeted biopsy. Using EUS, it is possible to arrange the mechanics of the instrument channel to ensure that a biopsy needle is accurately positioned within the target lesion (Figure 4-9). This has proven to be a technically complex task, but the necessary instruments are becoming commercially available. In the near future, it is likely that targeted biopsies using EUS will become quite sophisticated, with true core biopsies (single or multiple) being routinely obtained.

Three-Dimensional Endoscopic Ultrasound

Three-dimensional reconstruction of EUS images has been demonstrated by the Georgetown University group. Enhanced three-dimensional images

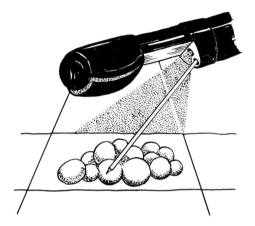

Figure 4-9. Radial scanning endoscopic ultrasound with angled biopsy channel through which an aspiration needle or injector can be passed.

of GI tract tumors will provide surgeons and radiation oncologists with valuable information needed for planning treatment. Presumably, Doppler flow information added to these images could detect vascular encasement and invasion, predicting operability (e.g., for pancreatic cancer). Three-dimensional EUS will also have a role in defining the structure of complex cysts, such as pancreatic pseudocysts.

Intraductal Ultrasound

Very thin ultrasound probes can be advanced into the biliary tree and pancreatic duct to provide unique images of the duct wall, including strictures and the surrounding tissues. It is fair to say that intraductal ultrasound remains a largely experimental tool. This technique may be particularly valuable in assessing bile duct and pancreatic duct strictures for malignancy and for detecting parenchymal abnormalities in pancreatitis, especially when the pancreatogram looks normal.

Training

Training in EUS is difficult to obtain because of the scarcity of opportunities for hands-on experience. The skills required to perform EUS are unique, and experience gained from standard endoscopy, including endoscopic retrograde cholangiopancreatography, is of limited benefit. To be a skilled practitioner of EUS one must acquire expertise in pattern recognition, an understanding of ultrasound and the nature of imaging artifacts, and the persistence to pursue the unknown. Considerable practice is necessary to become competent in this technique. The present generation of EUS experts learned by trial and error. Although a large and rapidly increasing body of literature now exists to guide the novice, it is still essential to gain hands-on supervised experience. It is possible that computer simulation and other related learning techniques will eventually allow beginners to practice their skills without recourse to patients, but these technologies are still in evolution. For the present, there is no substitute for the real thing. It is likely that prior training in transabdominal ultrasound will become a requirement for those learning EUS. Dr. Worth Boyce has addressed the need for a formal training syllabus in the *Proceedings of the Tenth International Symposium on Endoscopic Ultrasound.*

The number of EUS examinations required for competence is unknown. No data exist on which to base even a crude estimate. One of the world experts in the field has suggested that perhaps 75 examinations for abnormalities of the bowel wall and 200–250 EUS examinations for pancreatobiliary imaging would be required. Because the volume of EUS in many centers is quite low, trainees face a long apprenticeship. Until sufficient teachers of EUS emerge (and most are currently in training), there will be few opportunities to become expert in this technique. It is clear that the use of EUS will continue to expand as the technology is refined and more gastroenterologists become skilled in the technique.

Catalano et al. performed an interesting study of observer variation and reproducibility in EUS. They found that inexperienced EUS practitioners failed to agree on tumor (T) stage but did better with lymph node metastases (N). For experienced EUS operators, interobserver agreement was excellent for all T stages except T2. Agreement for N stage was excellent. The factors causing misinterpretation of T1 and T2 tumors are unknown but are the subject of continuing study.

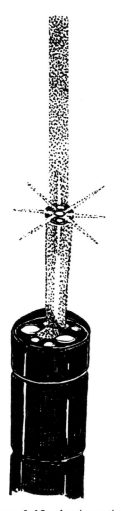

Figure 4-10. A schematic of a laser light guide emerging from an endoscopic instrument channel, with its laser beam heading off into the distance.

Lasers in Endoscopy

Although lasers are an undeniably attractive technology, they have been too expensive and too cumbersome to use routinely in our daily endoscopic practice (Figure 4-10). Cheaper and more easily applied methods for hemostasis of bleeding ulcers relegated medical lasers to dark corners of specialist centers, where they were used quite infrequently. As a result, those currently training in gastrointestinal endoscopy have few opportunities to work with lasers. My trainees frequently complain that information on the physics and tissue effects of laser energy is hard to find. This section attempts to remedy that situation, and provide some insights into the evolving uses of laser in the GI tract (Table 4-1).

A Short History of Laser

In 1913, the Danish physicist Niels Bohr, using quantum theory, overturned the classical Rutherford model of the atom. He was able to predict

Table 4-1. Common uses of laser in gastrointestinal endoscopy

Hemostasis
    Visible vessels
    Dieulafoy lesions
    Telangiectasia
    Watermelon stomach (gastric vascular ectasia)
    Friable tumors
Tumor ablation
    Recanalization of obstructed lumen esophagus
    Gastric cardia or antrum
    Colon or rectum debulking tumors (e.g., ampullary cancer), which cannot be resected for technical or patient health reasons
    Photodynamic therapy
Treatment of dysplasia (remains experimental)
    Barrett's esophagus
Optical biopsy
    To diagnose dysplasia and malignancy in accessible mucosal surfaces

with great accuracy the wavelengths of the emission spectra of hydrogen. The emission and absorption of light could now be explained by energy changes within atoms. These energy states, which are predicted by quantum theory, are restricted to allowable values only. These values depend on the configuration of orbiting electrons, which change from one energy state to another instantaneously. Such changes are accompanied by the absorption or emission of a packet of energy equal to the difference in energy between its two states, called the transitional energy. This packet of energy may be a photon (light). In molecules, a variety of discrete energy levels are present. These take the form of stretching and rotational vibrations of molecular bonds. Just as the energy states of a particular atom species are strictly defined, so also are the transition states of photon energies; i.e., an atom of any particular element can only emit or absorb photons of defined wavelengths and energies. Einstein showed that the release of a photon by an excited atom could occur not only spontaneously but by interaction with another photon of the correct energy. In this process, the incident photon remains unchanged and the newly emitted photon is identical to the incident one. This process of stimulated emission is the basis of the laser (*l*ight *a*mplification by *s*timulated *e*mission of *r*adiation).

Charles Townes, working for Bell Laboratories in the United States, and Nikolay Basov and Aleksandr Prokhorov of the Lebedev Institute in Moscow, independently realized that a photon emitted by an excited atom or molecule could, by initiating a chain of interactions with excited atoms or molecules of the same species, stimulate the emission of further identical photons. In 1951, Townes constructed the first *maser* (*m*icrowave *a*mplification by *s*timulated *e*mission of *r*adiation]. By 1958, Schwalow and Townes had worked out the conditions necessary for stimulated emission

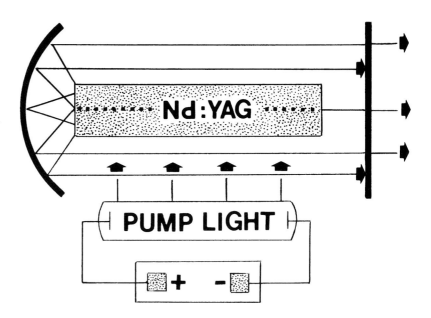

Figure 4-11. A neodymium-yttrium-aluminum-garnet crystal is primed to produce monochromatic laser light (exiting to the right) by photon bombardment (pump light). The laser light is amplified by a silvered (reflecting) surface and focused to produce a collimated beam by a convex mirror, represented by the curved line at the left end of the apparatus.

of optical and infrared wavelengths. The optical laser was renamed the LASER. The first working laser was constructed in 1960 by Thomas Maiman. In 1964, Townes, Basov, and Prokhorov shared the Nobel Prize in physics for the development of the laser.

Maiman created his laser using a small rod of synthetic ruby. Ruby is aluminum 203 with a small amount of chromium 304 held in a crystal lattice. Exciting the chromium^{3+} ions and letting them return to base energy level results in lasing. Maiman polished two faces of the ruby rod flat, then silvered them so that light traveling parallel to the long axis would be reflected back and forth. To allow light to escape, one end was left partially unsilvered (Figure 4-11). The energy needed to excite chromium^{3+} ions was provided by a gas discharge flash lamp. To further enhance the effect, the lamp was wound as a helix around the ruby and the whole device was sealed with a reflective coating. Without going into the complexities of the energy states of chromium^{3+}, the final step in the return to ground state results in pure, red laser light at 694 nm.

Development of the Neodymium-Yttrium-Aluminum-Garnet Laser

It was discovered in 1961 that the rare earth, neodymium (Nd), when doped in glass, had lasing properties. Neodymium is an excellent lasing medium because it has no less than four energy levels. The yttrium-aluminum-garnet (YAG) combination was found to be an effective host for the neodymium dope. To prime the laser, blue-green light emitted by a krypton lamp excites the trivalent neodymium ions into a band of high energy states, which then decay. Lasing occurs at the near-infrared wavelength of 1,064 nm. It is a common misconception that Nd:YAG laser light is visible, but it is the aiming beam, a helium-neon laser, that can be seen.

Argon Laser

It was suspected from theoretical considerations that gases could be lased. Helium was initially used as a buffer gas for the mercury laser. When helium became temporarily unavailable, argon was substituted. It was immediately noted that this enhanced the lasing effect. Indeed, the initial argon lasers proved so efficient that the tubes burnt out very quickly, due to high-energy ultraviolet light generated in the lasing process. It was not until 1972, when beryllium oxide tubes with quartz windows were developed, that it was possible to construct an argon laser in the 15- to 20-W energy range needed for medical applications.

Liquid Lasers

The first liquid lasers were demonstrated in 1966, when ruby laser light was used to excite solutions of dyes, such as chloroaluminum phthaloanaline. The wavelength of light emitted from certain dye lasers can be varied, giving rise to the tunable dye laser.

Resonator Cavities and Wave Guides

A variety of devices have been designed to enhance laser energy, including *resonator cavities*, which are parallel mirrors placed at a critical distance from each other. These allow a standing wave of laser light to form, producing an oscillation that greatly potentiates laser emission. Wave guides are specially coated optical fibers that internally reflect and transmit laser light with minimal losses. Wave guides are used to perform endoscopic laser treatment. The water-guided laser uses a stream of water to carry the laser energy. The water cools the target tissue to prevent vaporization when only coagulation is required.

Pulsed Lasers

By controlling the timing of laser pulses, higher-than-average energy pulses can be delivered in a noncontinuous form. Pulsed lasers have been used to fragment gallstones in the technique of laser lithotripsy.

Biological Effects of Laser

The tissue effects of laser depend on many factors, including wavelength, power, exposure time, beam characteristics, and the presence or absence of photosensitizing agents. The effects that a gastroenterologist needs to be aware of include the following:

- Thermal (vaporization, necrosis, coagulation)
- Photochemical and photodynamic
- Contact lithotripsy

The most important laser-tissue interactions are thermal. The laser delivers energy to tissue that is absorbed as heat. Three types of laser are currently used for their ability to transmit thermal energy: the carbon dioxide laser (wavelength, 10,600 nm in the far infrared), the Nd:YAG laser (wavelength, 1,064 nm in the near infrared), and the argon laser (wavelengths, 488 and 514 nm in the blue and green regions of the visible spectrum). The carbon dioxide laser is strongly absorbed by cellular water, whereas the Nd:YAG and argon lasers are preferentially absorbed by pigment. These absorption characteristics also determine the depth of penetration. At similar power, the carbon dioxide laser has an essentially surface effect (0.1 mm), whereas the argon laser penetrates 1 mm or so, and the Nd:YAG laser about 5 mm. The ultimate fate of laser-treated tissue falls into one of the following categories:

1. Total destruction
   a. Instant vaporization
   b. Necrosis, then sloughing
2. Destruction with reconstitution
   a. Necrosis, then healing by scarring
   b. Necrosis, then healing by regeneration
3. Reversible effects
   a. Edema and inflammation
   b. Local warming

Experience has shown that in the GI tract, the Nd:YAG laser is best for hemostasis. For well-defined targets, such as bleeding ulcer bases, hemostasis may be achieved with 0.5-second bursts of 50- to 80-W laser power. Up to 10 shots at this energy level appear to be safe in the stomach or duodenum when applied in a tight ring around the offending vessel. For tumor therapy, the laser power used is similar to that for bleeding (50–80 W), but the duration of the applications is longer (1–2 seconds), and many more shots are applied. Whereas treatment of a bleeding peptic ulcer might require a few hundred joules of laser energy, one session to treat an obstructing esophageal tumor might require 5,000–20,000 J.

Table 4-2. Differences between noncontact and contact lasers

Characteristics	Noncontact	Contact
Power used	High	Low
Power range (W)	60–100	10–30
Cost	Expensive	Less expensive
Precision	Fair	Excellent
Lateral scatter	Yes	Less
Tissue contact	None	Yes
Tip adherence	None	Yes
Smoke emission	High	Low

Source: Modified from N Krasner. Lasers in Gastroenterology. London: Chapman & Hall, 1991.

Contact Laser

Although noncontact (standoff) lasers are the standard for use in gastroenterology, a variety of contact probes have been developed for specialized indications (Table 4-2). Contact probes suffer from the disadvantage of adhesion of coagulum from treated tissue. This reduces their light-transmitting ability and therefore their effectiveness. Contact lasers, however, apply their energy more efficiently, so that much lower power is required to achieve tissue coagulation and vaporization. Most contact lasers have crystalline tips, often made from sapphire or artificial sapphire-like material. The tips can be shaped to provide windows or other mechanisms to direct and focus the laser energy.

Laser Training and Safety

Training

The use of lasers in gastroenterology requires appropriate training and supervised experience. Because none of the specialist endoscopy societies has issued specific guidelines about endoscopic laser training, many centers have developed their own. At Duke University, our gastroenterology fellows must attend a 3-hour laser orientation session before they are allowed to perform endoscopic laser therapy under supervision. The orientation includes an introduction to laser physics, laser-tissue interactions, laser safety, and clinical applications of laser in the GI tract. A bench demonstration shows the effect of various power settings and pulse durations of the Nd:YAG laser when applied to a piece of animal liver. A minimum of five supervised sessions using the Nd:YAG laser are required for certification of competence to treat bleeding lesions (ulcers, telangiectasia) and up to 20 sessions for palliation of obstructing tumors.

Table 4-3. Classification of lasers

Class I	Power not to exceed maximum permissible exposure for eye
Class II	Visible laser beam only; power up to 1 mW; eye protected by blink reflex of 0.25 seconds
Class III	
IIIa	Counts as Class II (to 5 W) provided that beam widened to allow blink reflex to protect eye
IIIb	Power up to 0.5 W; direct viewing hazardous
Class IV	Power over 0.5 W; extreme hazard

Laser Safety

The principal hazards of medical laser therapy are ocular injury and fire, although skin burns and smoke must also be considered. In a worst-case scenario, about 40% of Nd:YAG laser light entering the eye reaches the retina, and only 10% is absorbed. By contrast, the energy from a carbon dioxide laser penetrates only about 10–20 μm into the cornea. For this reason, the Nd:YAG laser presents more of an ocular safety hazard than the carbon dioxide laser. Laser physicists have developed maximum permissible exposure (MPE) levels for the eye. The MPE is calculated from the power of the laser, the duration of exposure, and the area exposed. Lasers are classified into four classes (I–IV) according to the hazard they present (Table 4-3). The total exposure of the retina to laser energy is limited by reflex blinking, which on average occurs in 0.25 seconds. It is also a function of the area of the pupil in a darkened room (about 0.4 cm^2). The total power of an Nd:YAG laser entering the pupil before a blink is approximately 1 mW, which is the power limit for class II lasers. Surgical lasers are usually in the class IV category; the helium-neon aiming beam of the Nd:YAG laser is class II.

Another concept developed for laser safety is the nominal ocular hazard distance, which defines how close the unprotected eye may approach the tip of the Nd:YAG laser light guide with safety. Assuming a power rating of 100 W (which is high), a beam divergence of 12 degrees, and an exposure duration of 1 second, the nominal ocular hazard distance is 5.6 meters.

Protective eyewear is necessary to protect the patient and operators from unintentional exposure to laser light. An optical filter is required to attenuate the laser light. For the Nd:YAG laser, the attenuation required is on the order of 30,000. For convenience, the attenuating power of laser eyewear is rated on a scale based on powers of 10. Some filters are strongly tinted green. Others allow most visible wavelengths through but strongly attenuate in the region of the Nd:YAG wavelength (1,064 nm). These goggles appear transparent. It is important that eyewear for use with lasers have side shields to prevent lateral exposure. Filters are available to cover the eyepiece of fiberoptic endoscopes. These are designed to deal with the phenomenon of flashback radiation, which at least theoretically can exceed the MPE.

Fire and explosion are potential dangers when lasers are used in the presence of combustible gases, as in the colon. Appropriate bowel preparation should avoid this. Smoke is produced when tissue is vaporized. A considerable volume of smoke can be generated during prolonged tumor ablation. A system to vent the smoke from the operating room or endoscopy suite makes life more pleasant for all concerned. Because there is risk of aerosol spread of papilloma viruses when treating warts (e.g., perineal, rectal, esophageal), masks capable of filtering viral particles should be worn during such procedures.

Designated Laser-Controlled Areas.   Where lasers are being used in the clinical setting, precautions must be taken to avoid unintended exposures. In addition to warning signs, measures must be taken to limit access to the treatment room when the laser is operating (i.e., bolting the door on the inside manually or automatically) or to ensure that protective eyewear is available outside the room (to be put on prior to entry). There are numerous additional safety recommendations that are beyond the scope of this discussion. A member of the hospital staff may be designated the Laser Safety Officer to ensure compliance with local and national laser safety standards.

Photodynamic Therapy

Patients with the inherited disorder porphyria have increased sensitivity to sunlight during attacks because of high levels of circulating porphyrins. These molecules, breakdown products of heme, absorb light. As far back as the 1940s, investigators reported that injected porphyrins increased tumor necrosis when the tumors were irradiated with light from a quartz lamp. In 1972, it was reported that glial tumors implanted subcutaneously in rats receiving hematoporphyrin were destroyed by light. Hematoporphyrin derivative injected intraperitoneally results in long-term cure from implanted tumors in mice and rats when illuminated by red light that can penetrate the abdominal wall.

The tissue effects of photodynamic therapy (PDT) depend on the uptake of chemicals by target cells (Figures 4-12 A–D). When illuminated by laser light of the appropriate wavelength, these chemicals undergo electrochemical changes that may result in fluorescence (useful for diagnosis) or the generation of reactive intermediates (e.g., singlet oxygen). These reactive molecules have a variety of biological effects, including cell injury and death by disrupting lipid membranes. The physics and chemistry of PDT are quite complex and beyond the scope of this brief review. Suffice it to say that PDT remains largely experimental at present. Early experience of PDT for obstructing esophageal cancer was not encouraging. Serious complications included massive tumor necrosis and tracheoesophageal fistula

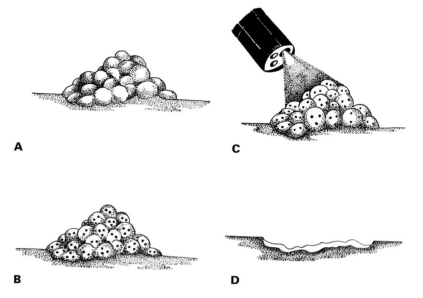

Figure 4-12. Photodynamic therapy (PDT): A. Abnormal tissue. B. Photosensitizing agent is taken up by abnormal tissue. C. Treated tissue is exposed to activating laser light. D. Treated tissue is killed by reactive metabolites of the photosensitizer and necroses.

formation. Other, less focused means of delivering the laser energy to the esophagus, such as placing the laser fiber in the center of a balloon filled with a light-dispensing medium, are being developed for clinical use. Small colonic tumors have been treated successfully with PDT. Delayed hemorrhage is a problem when larger colonic tumors are treated. For this reason, coagulation of the surface of the lesion using the Nd:YAG laser is recommended. Undoubtedly, the use of PDT will increase as photosensitizing agents and techniques for laser application are refined. There is considerable interest in the use of photosensitizing agents to detect and treat precancerous lesions of the GI tract, including Barrett's epithelium in the esophagus and dysplasia in the colon. Again, these applications remain experimental but hold great promise for the future.

Interstitial Laser Therapy

Current laser therapies for tumors are fairly crude. Fifty to 80 W of Nd:YAG laser power are routinely used to palliate advanced, obstructing tumors. Reducing the energy required to just a few watts would be a major advance. Interstitial laser therapy offers this prospect. Instead of delivering laser energy from a noncontact fiber or the tip of a contact probe, the fiber is inserted directly into the target. By this technique, the maximum response can be achieved anywhere within the target organ, with little observable effect at the surface. Of course, this means that the effect of the treatment cannot be determined by visual inspection alone. For interstitial laser therapy to be safe, it has to be monitored by some imaging technique, such as ultrasound. This is especially suitable for solid organs, such as liver and pancreas. Interstitial therapy is not without dangers. If the energy is delivered too fast, cellular water may vaporize and, being in a confined space, cause local disruption by pressure phenomena. Interstitial hyperthermia is carried out with laser power that is too low to cause vaporization (1–2 W), but other thermal effects occur, including necrosis. Exposure times are necessarily long (minutes or longer). Necrosis occurs up to 8–9 mm from the tip of the fiber, producing a necrotic zone up to 16–18 mm in diameter. This can be further enlarged using multiple fibers with overlapping treatment sites.

Suggested Reading

Enteroscopy

Chang J, Tagle M, Barkin JS, Reiner DK. Small bowel push-type fiberoptic enteroscopy for patients with occult gastrointestinal bleeding or suspected small bowel pathology. Am J Gastroenterol 1994;89:2147.

Lewis B, Waye J. Small bowel enteroscopy for obscure GI bleeding. Gastrointest Endosc 1991;37:277.

Yang R, Laine L. Mucosal stripping: a complication of push enteroscopy [editorial]. Gastrointest Endosc 1995;41:156.

Endoscopic Ultrasound

Catalano MF, Sivak MV Jr, Bedford RA, et al. Observer variation and reproducibility of endoscopic ultrasonography. Gastrointest Endosc 1995;41:115.

Furukawa T, Tsukamoto Y, Naitoli Y, et al. Differential diagnosis of pancreatic diseases with an intraductal ultrasound system. Gastrointest Endosc 1995;41:213.

Harada N, Kouzu T, Arima M, Isono K. Endoscopic ultrasound-guided histologic needle biopsy: preliminary results using a newly developed ultrasound transducer. Gastrointest Endosc 1996;44:327.

Hawes RH, Zaidi S. Endoscopic ultrasonography of the pancreas. Gastrointest Endosc Clin North Am 1995;5:61.

Kallimanis G, Garra BS, Tio TL, et al. The feasibility of three-dimensional endoscopic ultrasound: a preliminary report. Gastrointest Endosc 1995;41:235.

Proceedings of the 10th International Symposium on Endoscopic Ultrasonography. Gastrointest Endosc 1996;43(2, Suppl 2). (*Multiple authors; articles on the state of the art in endoscopic ultrasound technology.*)

Results of a Consensus Conference: clinical application of endoscopic ultrasonography in gastroenterology—state of the art 1993. Endoscopy 1993;25:359.

Saisho H, Sai K, Tsuyusuchi T, et al. A new small probe for ultrasound imaging via conventional endoscopes. Gastrointest Endosc 1995;41:141.

Savides TJ, Gress F, Sherman S, et al. Ultrasound catheter probe-assisted endoscopic cystogastrostomy. Gastrointest Endosc 1995;41:145.

Lasers in Endoscopy

Krasner N. Lasers in Gastroenterology. London: Chapman & Hall, 1991.

Pinkas H. Laser Therapy Update: ELT, PDT, LIF, Contact Probes, Low-Power Interstitial Sono-Guided Hyperthermia. In JS Barkin, CA O'Phelan (eds), Advanced Therapeutic Endoscopy (2nd ed). New York: Raven, 1994.

Photodynamic Therapy

Grosser L, Sroka R, Hahn EG, Ell C. Photodynamic therapy: successful destruction of gastrointestinal cancer after administration of aminolevulinic acid. Gastrointest Endosc 1995;41:55.

Raijman I, Lolar E, Marcon NE. Photodynamic therapy for tumor ingrowth through an expandable esophageal stent. Gastrointest Endosc 1995;41:73.

Index